To:

McIntyre family

[signature]

4/6/99.

A PRACTICAL ENCYCLOPEDIA

ACUPUNCTURIST'S HANDBOOK

KUEN-SHII TSAY, Lic. Ac., NCCA

Professor, Department of TCM

New England School of Acupuncture

A PRACTICAL ENCYCLOPEDIA

- Diagnosis Practicum • All Methods for Point Prescriptions • Basic and Advanced Techniques for Treatment • Scalp Acupuncture • Ear Acupuncture • Conceptions of Chinese Medicine

Revised and Expanded Edition

THE COMPLETE, PRACTICAL GUIDE TO THE DIAGNOSIS, POINT PRESCRIPTIONS, AND TECHNIQUES

ISBN-0-9647445-0-3

Library of Congress Catalog Card Number 95-069834

Production by

Pilgrim Type & Design
Plymouth, Massachusetts, USA

William S. Sullwold, Publishing
Taunton, Massachusetts, USA

Published by

CPM Whole Health
824 Boylston Street, Suite 100
Chestnut Hill, MA 02167 USA

DEDICATION

This book is dedicated in loving memory to my parents Minh and Shin Hsu Tsay. They were farmers who worked diligently and supported me while I attended Taipei Medical College in Taipei, Taiwan, R.O.C. Later, they sustained their faith and spirit in me when I attended Johns Hopkins University School of Medicine, Department of Clinical Pathology, in Baltimore, Maryland, U.S.A. My parents' inspiration and dedication lives on in the form of the Tsay Fellowship Award. This is the first and only award given to two outstanding graduate acupuncture students in the nation each year since 1991. It is presented by the New England School of Acupuncture in Watertown, Massachusetts.

Kuen-Shii Tsay
Newton, Massachusetts

ACKNOWLEDGMENTS

I would like to express my deepest appreciation to the following individuals who have provided interest, support, and their unique talents to the success of this project.

- Susan Kane, Lic. Ac., former faculty member at the New England School of Acupuncture in Boston, and Joshua Bellini, Lic. Ac., also a former faculty member at the New England School of Acupuncture, for their collaborative editorial efforts which deeply improved the clarity and accuracy of this manuscript.
- Laurie O'Brien, for her typing skills.
- Sonia E. Pantschenko, RN, for her extraordinary contributions, insights, and time.
- Lynda B. Norman, Lic. M.Th., and Christina Torode for creating balance in my demanding acupuncture practice, and coordinating the communication of those involved with this book.

Finally, to the readers of this book, I hope this text will serve you well in the special understanding and practice of acupuncture health care.

Kuen-Shii Tsay, Lic. Ac., NCCA
Professor, New England School of Acupuncture
CPM Whole Health-Tsay Acupuncture and Herbal Medicine
Newton, Massachusetts

PREFACE

The Acupuncturist's Handbook covers the complete, practical guide of the diagnosis, point prescriptions, techniques, scalp acupuncture, and ear acupuncture used in the clinical practice. The material is systematically presented with functions in an in-depth text. It is also a quick reference guide for acupuncture practitioners and students.

The book consists of three parts separated into twenty chapters. Each chapter is portrayed with detailed and descriptive explanations. Precise illustrations enable the practitioner to correctly perform the manipulation upon reading. Some of the material in this book has been presented at my lectures in acupuncture school since 1983.

This book is a compilation of diagnosis, point prescribing methods, and therapeutic procedures in a convenient pocket-size format which I feel to be of the greatest daily interest and value to the student and practitioner of acupuncture.

Kuen-Shii Tsay, Lic. Ac., NCCA
Professor, New England School of Acupuncture
Watertown, Massachusetts

PREFACE TO THE REVISED AND EXPANDED EDITION

Two editions of this book have been printed in the past two years. This text is intended to be a reference dictionary for both acupuncturists and acupuncture students. While producing this book, I have drawn freely upon the advice and criticism of many colleagues and students at the New England School of Acupuncture. The revised and expanded edition has been extensively reviewed with an addition of approximately 28 percent more information. New chapters and acupuncture concepts and illustrations of Chinese medicine have been added to create the most useful volume for acupuncture practice.

Kuen-Shii Tsay, Lic. Ac., NCCA

"This book is a wonderful book. I like the way that everything is set out so clearly. It seems like it will be a valuable clinical reference book for many people. I know that I will use it."
— *Acupuncturist in Massachusetts*

"I am sure this book will be of great use to me in my practice and in my teaching."
— *Faculty member of NESA*

"I recall your frustration in attempting to find a scholarly, complete and competently written textbook for your acupuncture students years ago. You vowed to write such a book when you could not locate one for your classes. With great success you have fulfilled your promise. Your textbook is certainly the most complete, intricate and thoughtfully written book on acupuncture today. It is a book for scholars and students to learn from and to keep as a reference book in their offices."
— *Acupuncturist in California*

CONTENTS

    A. Pulse ridge
    B. Five steps of finger movement
    C. Key pulses
    D. Eight principles and pulse types
    E. Methods of pulse diagnosis

    A. The seasons
    B. The Five Zang (solid) Organs
    C. Age
    D. Sex
    E. Physiological factors
    F. Other Conditions

    A. Superficial pulse
    B. Deep pulse
    C. Slow pulse

The General Process for Treatment of a Case with Acupuncture

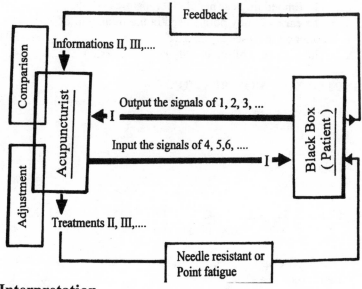

Interpretation

Gather and Interpret Information from the following three areas :

1. Medical Complaints (signaling the presence of symptoms)
2. Tender spots on the surface of the body (signaling the locations of diseases)
3. Pulse and tongue diagnosis (traditional Chinese medical diagnostics)
Other—Diagnostic Western Medical reports

Create a 3 Part Treatment Plan that addresses:

4. The Selection of Points (See page 105)
   a. Use of essential points
   b. Use of "Express" method
   c. Use of fewer points for less interference

5. The Needle Sensations
   Soreness, distension, numbness, cold, heat, pain.
   a. Excessive Syndrome: Numbness, distension, heat, and pain.
   b. Deficient Syndrome: Soreness, and cold.

6. Intensity and Time of Stimulation
   Strong, moderate, and weak.
   a. Acute, excessive syndromes: strong to moderate stimulation and
      shorter needle retention (less than 30 minutes).
   b. Chronic deficient syndromes: weak to moderate stimulation and
      longer needle retention (more than 30 minutes).
   Other— based on special clinical experience

Another perspective on the treatment process

If one imagines that the body is a "black box" of sorts that the Acupuncturist cannot open temporarily, and then one makes a detailed
study of the diagnostic signals (see 1, 2, and 3 above), or output, of
this "black box," one can then base the first treatment (see 4, 5, and 6
above), or input, on this study. Parts 4, 5, and 6 of this process should
be repeated at each treatment after the acupuncturist receives feed-
back from the patient, makes a comparison of the previous treatments
and results, and formulates adjustments necessary as a result of the
information received. Points can become needle resistant, or fatigued,
which will decrease their effectiveness. In order to derive the best
result from each treatment, one must avoid using the same points too
frequently, especially when the interval between successive treatments
is a short one.

The Conception of Treatment Process in Chinese Medicine Covers Both the Physical and Mental Aspects Simultaneously

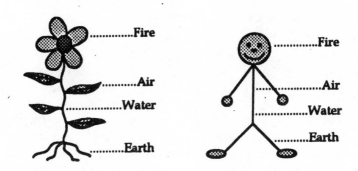

Interpretation

1. When one looks at the patient as a whole, one will see all their symptoms as parts of a bigger picture: a pattern.

2. When one organ in the body undergoes a pathological change, it will affect the functions of the other organs, which will be reflected in the physical and mental functions of the patient.

3. The human body, as shown in the chart, can be divided into four distinct parts, much as a flowering plant can be. These four parts correspond to the following elements as follows: Fire (the human head, the flower of the plant), Air (the human chest area, the leaves of the plant), Water (the human abdomen, the stem of the plant), and Earth (the four human limbs, the roots of the plant).

   This model suggests the following:
   a. The roots need earth in which to grow.
   b. The stem needs sufficient water in order to grow strong.
   c. The leaves need fresh air in order to sprout and be healthy.
   d. The flower needs enough food and water in order to become beautiful.

4. In essence, all the elements of an organism, human or plant, need to work together in order to heal disorders. The relationship of the elements of Earth, Air, Water, and Fire are critical to this healing process.

For example, a woman with a uterine fibroid tumor would have a disorder that would correspond in the four part system illustrated on this chart, to stagnation of qi in the Water area. This stagnation of water in her uterus, has allowed a pathological growth to occur. This is akin to a stagnant pond, which can become an ideal area for insects to grow. Thus we must incorporate the need to drain off this stagnant Water in the lower jiao, into our point prescription. We would devise a prescription that opened the Water area of the body and allowed the excess to drain into the Earth area, the clean air to flow through, clean out the growth, and vent the smoke (tension and stress) out the Fire area of the body (the upper jiao). This last is akin to a firefighter opening the windows of a burning house to vent out the smoke.

Most patients with chronic or persistent disorder experience some degree of tension, stress, and depression. Therefore, in order to obtain the best results from each treatment, our treatment principles, and points selection must address this. We must utilize points from the different meridians involved with the disorder, points that address both the physical and mental components of the disorder, if we are to help all parts of the body to work together in the healing process.

The Grant Qi Circulatory System

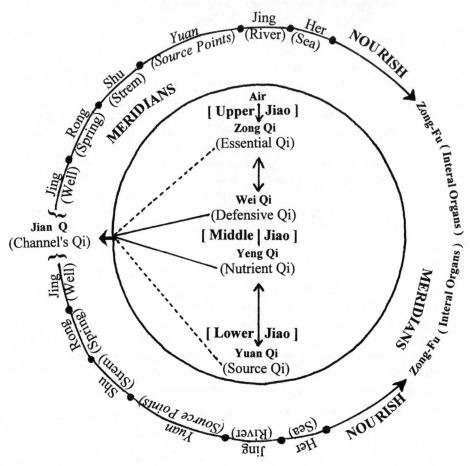

Interpretation

The Grant Qi circulatory system consists of Source Qi, Channel's Qi, Nutrient Qi, Defensive Qi and Essential Qi.

▼ Inherited from parents

1. **Yuan Qi** (Source Qi or congenital Qi) ⟶pass through Sanjiao (lower, middle and upper jiao) ⟶flourishes Five Shu Points ⟶retains Source Points (Yuan Points) ⟶meets with Acquired Channel's Qi ⟶nourishes Internal Organs for reproductive function.

▼ From the part of nutrient Qi

2. **Jian Qi** (channel's Qi or functional Qi) $\xrightarrow{\text{circulates}}$ From the terminals of the extremities to internal organs $\xrightarrow{\text{nourishes}}$ Internal organs.

▼ From the essential substance in food

3. **Yen Qi** (nutrient Qi or substantial Qi) $\xrightarrow{\text{corresponds to}}$ RBC (red blood cell) and protein $\xrightarrow{\text{nourishes}}$ Internal organs.

▼ From the essential substance in food

4. **Wei Qi** (defensive Qi or substantial Qi) $\xrightarrow{\text{corresponds to}}$ WBC (white blood cell), macrophages, monocytes and lymphocytes $\xrightarrow{\text{defend}}$ body against exogenous pathogenic factors.

▼ From air (oxygen) and food

5. **Zong Qi** (essential Qi or substantial Qi) $\xrightarrow{\text{accumulating in}}$ Chest, stomach and liver $\xrightarrow{\text{dominates}}$ Nutrient and defensive Qi $\xrightarrow{\text{nourishes}}$

    a. Heart for blood circulatory function
    b. Lung for respiratory function

The Balanced Principle of the Relative Amounts of Qi and Blood in the 12 Meridians – See page 187

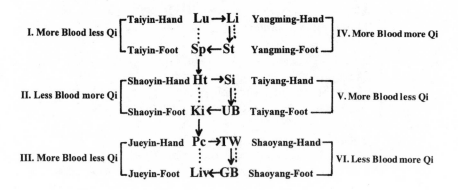

Interpretation

1. ──▶ Connected meridians
   . . . . . Connected same name of meridians

2. More (+), Less (-)

3. ↕ Zang (solid) organs
   a. I (more Blood less Qi) + II (less Blood more Qi)
      I + II = (+ Blood - Qi) + (- Blood + Qi) = 0 (Balance)
   b. II (less Blood more Qi) + III (more Blood less Qi)
      II + III = (- Blood + Qi) + (+ Blood - Qi) = 0 (Balance)

   ↕ Fu (hollow) organs:
   a. IV (more Blood more Qi) + V (more Blood less Qi)
      IV + V = (+ Blood + Qi) + (+ Blood - Qi) = 2 (Blood)
   b. V (more Blood less Qi) + VI (less Blood more Qi)
      V + VI = (+ Blood - Qi) + (- Blood + Qi) = 0 (Balance)

4. ↔ Zang & Fu Organs:
    a. I (more Blood less Qi) + IV (more Blood more Qi)
        I + IV = (+ Blood - Qi) + (+ Blood + Qi) = <u>2 (Blood)</u>
    b. II (less Blood more Qi) + V (more Blood less Qi)
        II + V = (- Blood + Qi) + (+ Blood - Qi) = <u>0 (Balance)</u>
    c. III (More Blood less Qi) + VI (less Blood more Qi)
        III + VI (+ Blood - Qi) + (- Blood + Qi) = <u>0 (Balance)</u>

Thus,

Up and down = Left and right

$$\updownarrow \quad = \quad \longleftrightarrow \qquad \qquad \longleftrightarrow\!\updownarrow \; = \textbf{ Balance}$$

2 (Blood)   2 (Blood)

The 12 Meridians of hands and feet are connected to each other to make Qi and Blood circulation in the whole body

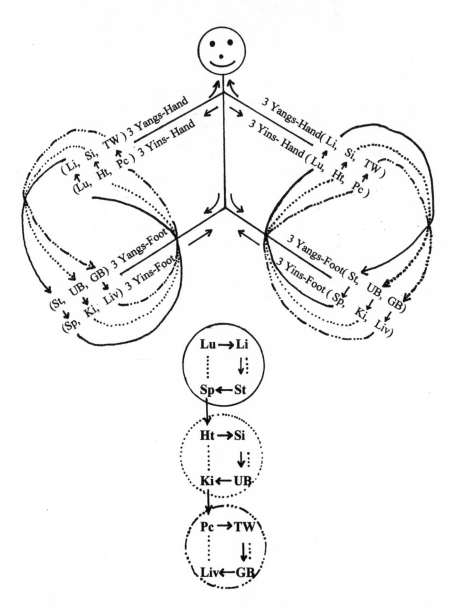

PART ONE

DIAGNOSIS PRACTICUM

Chapter I

Pulse Diagnosis

CHAPTER I.   PULSE DIAGNOSIS

Pulse diagnosis is an integral aspect of Chinese medicine. It is used by the practitioner to understand pathological changes taking place and to identify the syndrome in each case.

CONCEPTS

A. Pulse Ridge

Each pulse has an area in the center known as the "pulse ridge". The pulse is felt with three fingers: the index, middle and ring fingers. The pad of the fingertip , or the "finger eye", is placed on the pulse ridge for taking the pulse. The fingers should be flexed and relaxed much like the hands of a pianist.

B. Five Steps of Finger Movement

There are five basic movements to be made in feeling the pulse quality.

1. Up and down: the fingers move up and down in position to determine if the pulse is superficial or deep.

2. Right and left: the fingers move right and left or side-to-side to establish whether the pulse is long or short.

3. Push and seek: the fingers are feeling for the breadth of the pulse, whether wide or thin, as well as the strength of the pulse, be it "Xu" (deficient) or "Shi" (excessive).

4. Holding the pulse: the fingers are held on the pulse region for several moments in order to determine if the rate is slow or rapid and whether the quality is "rolling" ("slippery") or wiry".

5. Moving the fingers singly or together: one finger can be held in its position or all three fingers can be moved at once to determine if the pulse is regular or irregular in its rhythm.

C. Key Pulses

There are three key pulses that pertain to different energetic functions. These pulses are the Wei pulse, the Shen pulse and the Ken pulse.

1. The Wei pulse (Stomach pulse)

> The Wei pulse corresponds to the Qi of the stomach. The stomach is the source of health. The Wei pulse is located in the second position at the wrist which corresponds to the Middle Warmer. The Wei pulse should be neither superficial nor deep, nor should it be rapid or slow. This pulse should be even and forceful with a regular rhythm.

2. The Shen pulse (Heart pulse)

> In Chinese medicine, it is said that the Heart houses the Mind. A healthy person has good mental faculties such as memory, consciousness, reasoning and spirit. The Shen pulse reveals the quality of the mind and spirit. A normal Shen pulse will be peaceful and without weakness.

3. The Ken pulse (Kidney pulse)

> The Kidney stores the Essential Qi, or Jing Qi. The Kidney also functions to receive Qi and govern reproduction, growth and development. The Kidney Qi in the body is like the root system of a tree. A normal Kidney pulse is deep and forceful.

D. Eight Principles and Pulse Types

Eight Principles	Pulse Types
YIN	DEEP AND SLOW
YANG	SUPERFICIAL AND RAPID
EXTERIOR	SUPERFICIAL AND FORCEFUL

INTERIOR	DEEP AND WEAK
COLD	SLOW
HEAT	FAST
DEFICIENCY	WEAK
EXCESS	FORCEFUL

E. Methods of Pulse Diagnosis

The patient should be relaxed and comfortable while his pulse is being taken. Ask him to rest for five to ten minutes in a chair or on the treatment table before the pulses are taken. This allows the Qi to become peaceful and the circulation to flow smoothly in the pulse region. Let the patient extend his arm in a relaxed manner with the palm upward.

The acupuncturist should first place his middle finger on the interior side of the styloid process of the radius and then place the second and fourth fingers above and below it respectively. The second finger is on the CUN region of the pulse; the middle finger is on the GUAN region; the fourth finger is on the CHI region. If the patient is a small person, the acupuncturist will need to place his fingers more closely together; if the patient is a large person, the fingers will be further apart.

The acupuncturist should be relaxed while taking the pulse. His mind should be peaceful and focused in order to feel the three pulse regions and make comparisons. There are three degrees of pressure, or "finger force", to apply when feeling a pulse: mild or slight, moderate and heavy. These different degrees of pressure are applied while using the five finger movements described earlier in this chapter. If the pulse responds to the fingers when pressed lightly, it is a Yang pulse and it reflects the condition of the Heart and Lung. If the pulse can be felt when pressed moderately, it is a Yin pulse reflecting the Qi of the Liver and Kidney. If the pulse can only be felt when pressed heavily, it is indicative of the Spleen and Stomach.

THE NORMAL PULSE

Although a healthy person will have a "normal" pulse, there are several factors which effect the form of a normal pulse such as the seasons, physiological function, age, sex, the body's constitution, and environmental factors. The following is a list of these correspondences:

FACTOR   PULSE QUALITY

A. The Seasons

The normal pulse takes on different characteristics as the seasons change.

Spring   deep, rolling (slippery) and long

Summer   superficial, wiry and wide

Autumn   superficial, rough and short

Winter   deep, thin and smooth

B. The Five Zang (Solid) Organs

Heart   superficial, wide and wiry

Lung   superficial, rough and short

Kidney   deep, thin and smooth

Liver   deep, rolling (slippery) and long

Spleen   superficial, rough and wide

C. Age

child   thin, rolling (slippery) and rapid; the younger
                            the child, the more rapid the pulse.

adult (20 - 40 years) wiry, wide and long; this pulse indicates good physical strength. In some healthy adults, the pulse is either deep and thin or rapid and wide: both forms of pulses indicate normal physiological function in a healthy adult.

elder (60+ years old) deep and weak; the quality of the Qi and the strength of the circulation of blood are both waning with age.

D. Sex

male   superficial and wide

female   deep and thin

fetal sex: male   the mother's pulse in the Chi region of the left hand will be wide and rapid; the Cun regions of both hands will be slippery.

fetal sex: female   the mother's pulse in the Chi region of both hands will be wide, rapid and slippery.

E. Physiological Factors

obesity   deep, thin and long (due to looseness of the musculature).

thin   superficial and short

menses   a few days before the onset of menstrution each cycle, the Guan and Chi pulse regions suddenly become wide.

pregnancy   during the first trimester, the pulse in the Cun region of the left hand as well as the pulse of the Chi regions of both hands is slippery and rapid.

F. Other Conditions

after eating   wide and slow

when hungry   weak

after drinking alcohol   wide and rapid

walking long distances   rapid

THE CLINICAL SIGNIFICANCE OF
THE SIXTEEN COMMON PULSES

A. Superficial Pulse

The superficial pulse can be felt when pressed lightly. It becomes weak with heavy pressure. This pulse usually occurs in exterior syndromes.

1. Superficial and forceful

    This is an Exterior and Excess syndrome. It is associated with Heat or Yang syndromes. The patient will have fever but no sweating.

2. Superficial and forceless

    This is an Exterior and Deficient syndrome that is associated with a Yin Syndrome. The patient will have fever with sweating

The superficial and forceless pulse is also indicative of a Yin Deficient syndrome with symptoms of dry mouth, red tongue proper and heat in the palms of the hands and the soles of the feet.

B. Deep Pulse

The deep pulse can only be felt when pressed heavily. This pulse usually appears in Interior syndromes. The patient will show symptoms such as cold hands and feet, pain in the joints, edema, difficulty in raising arms, stasis of blood, and diarrhea. The deep pulse is differentiated by its relative strength or weakness.

1. Deep and forceful

   This pulse indicates an Interior and Excess syndrome such as Stagnation of Qi and Blood.

2. Deep and forceless

   This pulse indicates an Interior and Deficient syndrome such as Deficiency of the Yang Qi.

If the deep pulse is found in a patient who has an Exterior syndrome with a fever, it indicates that the functioning of both the heart and the nervous system are very weak. Another configuration that indicates very poor functioning of the nervous system is the superficial pulse with an Interior syndrome. Both of these cases indicate a severe and dangerous condition.

C. Slow Pulse

The pulse rate of the slow pulse is less than four beats per respiration. It usually occurs in Cold syndromes of a deficient nature. If the slow pulse appears in a patient who has Deficient Yang Qi, it indicates that the patient suffers from weak functioning of the heart.

1. Slow and forceful

   This pulse is characteristic of Cold syndromes and is associated with pain.

2. Slow and forceless

   This pulse is associated with Cold and Deficient syndromes.

A slow pulse in the presence of a Heat syndrome is indicative of mental disorders such as depression and anxiety.

D. Rapid Pulse

The rapid pulse has a rate of more than five beats per respiration. This pulse usually occurs in patterns of Heat, hyperactivity of Yang Qi, and Deficient Yin syndromes.

1. Rapid and forceful

   This pulse is found in Excessive Heat syndromes as well as in hyperactivity of the Yang Qi, such as an exogenous disorder with cold and heat, dryness, thirst, phlegm heat, blood in the stool, and furuncle.

2. Rapid and forceless

   The rapid pulse that is without strength indicates a Deficient Yin syndrome and prolonged illness with Yin Deficiency.

E. Xu (Deficient) Pulse

The Xu pulse is weak and forceless when pressed lightly and it becomes an empty pulse when pressed heavily. This pulse often occurs in deficient syndromes such as Deficiency of both of Qi and Blood, dysfunction of the lung, excessive sweating, weakness in the legs, and indigestion.

1. Wide and has no peaceful and forceful indicates Yin Deficiency.

2. Thin and has no peaceful and forceful: Yang deficiency.

F. Shi (Excessive) Pulse

The pulse is still responsive to the finger even on deep pressure. It is forceful, big and long. The Shi pulse usually occurs in excessive syndromes such as Stagnation of the Qi, Interior attack of the heat, constipation, and indigestion.

1. Shi (excessive) and even quality

The Shi pulse that is peaceful and even indicates that the body has enough vital energy.

2. Shi (excessive) but without even quality

If the Shi pulse is found in the presence of a Deficiency syndrome and after sweating, diarrhea, and hemorrhage following labour, it indicates that the patient is suffering from vascular sclerosis.

G. Rolling (slippery) Pulse

The rolling, or slippery, pulse is called Yang Pulse. It has a smoothly flowing and forceful quality to it. It usually occurs in conditions of excessive phlegm, nausea and vomiting, cough, stasis of the blood, abdominal distention, and diarrhea.

In a person who has enough Wei (defensive) Qi and Yeng (nutrient) Qi, the pulse will be rolling. If a healthy woman has a rolling pulse, it could indicate pregnancy.

H. Rough Pulse

The rough pulse feels uneven when palpated. It is described as being like a knife shaving bamboo. It is the opposite of a rolling pulse. It usually occurs in syndromes of Insufficiency of the Blood, Insufficiency of the Qi, Bi Syndrome, Cold Damp, diarrhea, seminal emission in the men, and lost blood in women.

If the rough pulse occurs in the patient with the symptoms of intolerance to cold, vomiting and diarrhea, cold in the four limbs, sweating, the absence of thirst, and a white tongue coating, it is a Cold syndrome.

If the rough pulse occurs in the patient with the symptoms of fever with sweating, abdominal distention, insufficiency of blood, constipation, anxiety, thirst, and a red tongue proper, it is a Heat syndrome.

I. Wiry Pulse

The wiry pulse is forceful, straight and tight. It usually occurs in Liver disorders, pain disorders, Deficient Blood syndromes, Wind Phlegm, malaria, abdominal pain and pain in the lateral side of the chest. A wiry, thin and forceful pulse indicates a severe condition in which the Stomach Qi is very weak.

J. Thin (Small) Pulse

The thin pulse can be felt easily but it is like a fine thread. It often occurs in Deficiency of Blood and Qi, Deficient syndromes, and Damp syndromes.

If a person without illness has a thin and weak pulse, it indicates the Insufficiency of Source (Yuan) Qi in the body.

If a thin pulse appears in a Heat or Excessive syndrome, it indicates a severe condition.

K. Short Pulse

The short pulse is uneven in movement, is of short duration, and does not fill the pulse region. This pulse is usually found in Stagnation of the Qi, Deficiency of Blood, Deficiency of Lung Qi, indigestion, and impaired circulation. The short pulse, for example, may be present in a patient who has anemia with headaches.

1. Short and forceful

    This pulse indicates Stagnation of Qi.

2. Short and forceless

    This pulse indicates impairment of Qi.

3. Short and rapid

    This pulse indicates a serious heart disorder.

L. Long Pulse

The long pulse can be felt clearly over the length of the pulse region. The difference between the long pulse and the wiry pulse is that the long pulse is slower and smoother than the wiry pulse.

The long pulse usually occurs in Excessive syndromes such as hyperactivity of Fire, Heat in the Triple Warmer Meridian (Sanjiao), Interior Retention of the pathogenic Yang Qi, and Stomach Heat.

1. Long, slow and peaceful

    This pulse indicates a healthy condition with sufficient Qi.

2. Long, wiry and forceful

    This pulse indicates the hyperactivity of the Liver Yang and an Interior Heat syndrome.

M. Wide Pulse

The wide pulse is felt to be big and spreading under the fingers. This pulse is often found in Excessive Heat syndromes and it is associated with anxiety and upset, thirst, hemoptysis, and abdominal distention. It can also reflect a Yin Deficiency with hyperactivity of Yang Qi. If the wide pulse is present in a patient suffering from prolonged disease and fatigue, the patient's condition is grave.

1. Wide and forceful

    Pathogenic Qi is accumulating.

2. Wide and forceless

    The pathogenic Qi is declining.

N. Tight Pulse

The tight pulse is big, wiry and long and it responds to the finger under heavy pressure. This pulse is indicates Interior Excessive Cold and Yin syndrome as well as Interior Stagnation of Qi. This pulse never occurs in deficient syndromes. If this pulse appears in the presence of hemorrhage or Yin Deficiency, it is a severe case.

O. Knotted Pulse

The knotted pulse is a slow pulse with an irregular pattern of missed beats. It often occurs in Stagnation of Qi with retention of Cold Phlegm, disharmony of Yin and Yang with endogenous Cold, Stasis of Blood, and in cases of chronic illness and weakness. If the knotted pulse suddenly appears in a healthy person, it indicates a cardiac valve disorder.

P. Intermittent Pulse

The intermittent pulse is a slow pulse with a pattern of long gaps between sets of beats. It usually occurs in syndromes of weakness of the Qi of the internal organs, Wandering Bi syndrome, and impairment of Qi and Blood due to physical injury. This pulse occasionally occurs in pregnant women.

THE DIFFERENTIATION OF THE PULSE

A. The Six Major Pulses Dominating Other Pulses

Pulse Description	Associated Pulses	Clinical Indications
Superficial pulse	wide pulse wiry pulse	Exterior syndrome
Deep pulse	tight pulse	Interior syndrome
Slow pulse	rough pulse knotted pulse intermittent pulse	Cold syndrome
Rapid pulse	tight pulse	Heat syndrome
Xu pulse	thin pulse short pulse weak pulse	Deficient syndrome
Shi pulse	long pulse rolling or slippery pulse	Excessive syndrome

B. Pulse Regions and Clinical Indications

Pulse Description	Pulse Position	Clinical Indications
wiry pulse	the Guan region of the left hand	Liver disorders
weak pulse	the Cun region of the left hand	Lung disorders

The clinical manifestations of the heart, liver, and kidney are reflected respectively in the Cun, Guan and Chi positions of the left hand. The right hand reflects the condition of the lungs, spleen and kidney in the Cun, Guan and Chi positions.

A disorder of a specific organ is indicated when the pulses in the Cun, Guan and Chi regions are the same:

Pulse Description	Organ Disorder
Superficial pulse	Lung
Deep pulse	Kidney
Wide pulse	Heart
Wiry pulse	Liver
Slow pulse	Spleen

C. Pulses that are Inconsistent with the Syndromes

In severs syndromes, the pulse may reflect combinations of qualities that seem inconsistent.

Pulse Quality	Normal Indication	Other Pulse Qualities	Clinical Indication
superficial	Exterior syndrome	weak forceless	Yin Deficiency Deficient Blood Impaired Qi
deep	Interior syndrome	tight	Exogenous Cold
rapid	Heat	extremely rapid	Severe deficiency syndrome with disharmony of both Qi and Blood
slow	Cold	slippery	The patient is just recovering from exogenous disorder; Heat remains in the body
wiry and forceful	Excess	wide	Deficiency of Stomach Fire
thin	Deficiency	wiry	Stagnation of Qi with severe pain

D. Contradictions in Pulse Readings

Occasionally, different pulse qualities can be perceived in the course of taking the pulse for a minute or two.

Pulse Description	Indication
First impression is superficial and wide and second impression is weak and thin	An extreme deficiency with deficient Yang flaring up to cause a superficial and wide pulse
First impression is weak and second impression is forceful	An Interior syndrome without impairment of the Qi of the internal organs
First impression is slightly weak and slightly wiry and the second impression is slow and peaceful	The patient is recovering from a prolonged illness; there is Deficiency of both Qi and Blood but the internal organ function is good
First impression is smooth and peaceful and the second impression is weak, or wiry and no longer responds to heavy finger pressure	A severe condition

Chapter II

Palpation of the Body and Meridians

CHAPTER II. PALPATION OF THE BODY AND MERIDIANS

The application of both hands on the body of the patient assists the practitioner in recognizing the pathological changes taking place.

A. Superficial Palpation

The palpation of the surface of the body enables the practitioner to determine areas of abnormally cold or hot temperatures. The perception of increased surface temperature of the body indicates a Heat syndrome and the hyperactivity of pathogenic Qi. The perception of cold areas of the surface of the body points to a Cold syndrome and a decline in the strength of the Yang Qi.

Mild Pressure

Method: the hands press lightly on the surface of the body and a strong heat area is felt; with deeper and for longer pressure, this heat becomes normal

Indication: Exterior Heat
Heat in the Lung
Deficient Heat due to physical exhaustion

Moderate Pressure

Method: Heat is felt with moderate pressure; it becomes normal upon deeper pressure

Indication: Interior Heat in the Middle Jiao (Spleen and Heart)

Heavy Pressure

Method: heavy pressure to the tendons and bone reveals the presence of strong heat

Indication: Deficient Yin
Damp Heat

B. Palpation of the Hands and Feet

The purpose of palpation of the hands and feet is to determine the presence of a Cold or Heat syndrome and the strength of the Yang Qi of the body.

A. In Adult:

Region	Palpation Diagnosis	Indication
Hands and feet	cold during the onset of disease	Yin Cold; slower recovery from illness
Hands and feet	warm	recovers from llness easily
Back of hand	strong heat	exogenous disorder; Wind Cold
Palm of hand	strong heat	endogenous disorder

B. In children:

Palms of hands	heat	heat syndrome
	cold	severe condition
Feet	cold	cold syndrome
Tips of fingers	cold	convulsion
Middle finger	cold	Wind Cold

C. Palpation of the Chest and Abdomen

The chest and abdomen house the internal organs referred to as the Five Zang (solid) and the Six Fu (hollow) organs. This is the region of the origin of Qi and Blood. It is also the area where a disease pathogen may enter and develop in the body. Palpation of the chest and abdomen facilitates the differential diagnosis of an Exterior or Interior syndrome, an Excess or Deficient syndrome, and a Cold or Heat syndrome.

1. The moistness of the skin can be assessed by light palpation of the abdomen. Dryness indicates a Heat syndrome while a clammy quality indicates a Cold syndrome.

2. Tenderness or pain upon moderate and repeated pressure to the muscles indicates the accumulation of pathogenic Qi.

3. Softness or hardness of the muscles upon palpation with heavy pressure indicates a Deficient or Excess syndrome respectively of the internal organs as well as the development of pathogenic Qi.

Palpation of the Chest

There are two areas on the chest that are significant for palpation.

1. The area that is one rib below the nipple of the left breast, or between the fourth and fifth ribs, is called the Xu Li spot.

   a. In a normal condition, the heart beat feels forceful and smooth; it is not rapid or tight.

   b. A heartbeat that is weak and indistinct, indicates the Interior Deficiency of Qi.

   c. A heartbeat that is so strong that it can be seen on the skin indicates hyperactivity of the Qi.

2. The area inferior to the heart and below the xyphoid process is palpated to determine whether there is Stagna-

tion of Qi in the Upper or Middle Jiao (chest and abdominal area).

    a.   Distention, hardness and tenderness in this area indicates chest fullness or severe indigestion.

    b.   Distention without tenderness in this area indicates Insufficient Yin of the Lung due to endogenous Heat.

Palpation of the Abdominal region

The abdominal region is palpated for signs of distention, tenderness and pain. Distention and tenderness in the abdominal region indicates the Interior Retention of Damp in the Upper or Middle Jiao.

1. <u>Distention and Swelling</u>

If the abdomen is distended and tender upon palpation, an Excess syndrome is present. An abdomen that is distended but not sensitive to pressure suggests a Deficient syndrome.

If the abdomen sinks when pressure is applied and does not return to its normal condition when the fingers are lifted, then the condition is one of severe water retention or ascites.

When the distended abdomen is pressed and it does return to its normal state after pressure, the distention is due to the retention of air and the Stagnation of Qi.

2. <u>Tenderness and Pain</u>

The symptom of sharp pain from lower part of the abdominal region which spreads to the genital area upon palpation and is associated with a rapid and tight pulse indicates acute enteritis.

The symptom of dull, fixed pain that is located in the lower part of the abdomen and accompanies a slow and wide pulse indicates chronic enteritis.

D Palpation of the Forehead

The palpation of the forehead assists the acupuncturist in diagnosing the condition of a child.

If the child has a Deficient Heat condition, the palms of the hands will be warmer than the forehead.

If the child has an Excess Heat condition, the forehead will be hotter than the palms of the hands.

E. Palpation of the Meridians

The Back-Shu Points

The Back-Shu points are located on the medial line of the Urinary Bladder Channel where the Qi of the respective internal organs is infused. These points have an important role in diagnosis. Whenever there is a dysfunction any of the internal organs, the associated Back-Shu points will become tender.

Back-Shu Point:	Associated Organ:
UB 13 (Fei Shu)	Lung
UB 15 (Xin Shu)	Heart
UB 18 (Gan Shu)	Liver
UB 19 (Dan Shu)	Gall Bladder
UB 20 (Pi Shu)	Spleen
UB 21 (Wei Shu)	Stomach
UB 23 (Shen Shu)	Kidney
UB 25 (Da Chang Shu)	Large Intestine
UB 27 (Xiao Chang Shu)	Small Intestine
UB 28 (Pangguang Shu)	Urinary Bladder

The Yuan (Source) Points

The Yuan (Source) points for each of the 12 meridians have a great significance in diagnosis and treatment. Abnormal tenderness with palpation of the Yuan (Source) points indicates pathological changes in its associated organ.

Yuan (Source) Point:		Associated Organ:
Lu 9	(Tai Yuan)	Lung
L.I. 4	(He Gu)	Large Intestine
St 42	(Chung Yang)	Stomach
Sp 3	(Tai Bai)	Spleen
Ht 7	(Shen Men)	Heart
S.I. 4	(Wang Gu)	Small Intestine
Ki 3	(Tai Xi)	Kidney
UB 64	(Jing Gu)	Urinary Bladder
Pc 7	(Da Ling)	Pericardium
TW 4	(Yang Chi)	Triple Warmer
GB 40	(Qiu Xu)	Gall Bladder
Liv 3	(Tai Chong)	Liver

F. Palpation of the Spinal Nerves

The peripheral nervous system consists of thirty-one pairs of seg-
mentally arranged spinal nerves that connect the spinal cord to the
various parts of the body. There are eight cervical nerves, twelve thoracic nerves, five lumbar nerves, five sacral nerves and one coccygeal
nerve. A tender spot appearing in any pair of spinal nerves is associated with dysfunction of the corresponding internal organ.

Nerve Segment:	Associated Region of the Body:
C1-C8	head and face
T1-T3	heart
T1-T4	upper limbs
T2-T5	lung
T5-T8	stomach
T8-T10	liver
T10-T12	kidney
T12-L2	intestines
L1-L4	lower limbs
sacral and coccygeal nerves	genital organs

Chapter III

Tongue Diagnosis

CHAPTER III. TONGUE DIAGNOSIS

The condition of the Zang organs is revealed by examination of the tongue. The different areas of the tongue are related to the organs of Spleen, Kidney, Liver, Heart, and Lung.

Yin is associated with physical strength or vigor. It is an inner quality and it is reflected in the tongue. Yang is associated with the spirit, or Shen. Yang qualities refer to emotional states and to life style. It is an outer quality that reveals itself on the face in the six Yang meridians, the Conception Vessel (CV) and the Governing Vessel (GV).

CONCEPTS

A. Normal Tongue Proper

The tongue is a muscle that connects to the upper parts of the pharynx and larynx which connect to the trachea and lung. The normal color of the body of the tongue is light red. The tongue must also have normal movement to it, that is, it should be neither stiff nor quivering.

B. Normal Tongue Coating

A normal tongue will have a thin white coating that is moist.

The clinical diagnosis of the tongue proper is more significant than the tongue coating.

C. Seven Steps of Tongue Diagnosis

The tongue should be examined for seven parameters.

1. the color of the tongue proper (see page 32)

2. the tip of tongue (red spots on the tip of the tongue indicate a Heat syndrome even though the tongue coating may be white)

3. the center of tongue: the absence of a tongue coating indicates a Yin Deficiency.

4. the moisture on the tongue proper: a dry tongue indicates a Deficiency of essential fluid.

5. the borders of the tongue:

    a. if the tongue coating on both of borders is thick but there is no coating on the surface of the tongue it indicates that a pathogenic factor has attacked the interior organs but it is not a serious condition.

    b. if the tongue coating is thick on the surface of the tongue, but it is absent from the border of the tongue it indicates that the interior pathogenic factor is becoming weak and the condition will show improvement

6. the root of the tongue (in syndromes of Yin Deficiency, the tongue coating is not always connected to the root of the tongue)

7. the tongue coating (see page 34)

THE DIFFERENTIAL DIAGNOSIS OF THE TONGUE PROPER

There are three categories of tongue color to differentiate: pale, deep red, and purplish.

A. Pale Tongue Proper

1. Deficiency of both Qi and Blood

The tongue is pale in color. The size of the tongue is normal or smaller than normal and it is not flabby or swollen. The surface of the tongue is moist without excessive fluid. The clinical signs in this syndrome are low voice, shallow respiration, spontaneous sweating, palpitations, dizziness, ringing in the ears, and pale lips. The pulse is weak and thin, or intermittent.

2. Yang Deficiency and Damp Cold

The tongue is pale, flabby, and wet. The border of the tongue has scalloped indentations, or teeth prints. The clinical signs of this syndrome are intolerance to cold, cold in the four limbs, edema, loose bowel movement and fatigue. The pulse is deep and slow.

B. Deep Red Tongue Proper

1. Excess Heat

With the onset of febrile diseases, the color of the tongue becomes a deep, bright red. The pathogenic Heat is hyperactive and the vital Qi is weak. In the advanced stage of febrile disease, the deep red color is prominent and the surface of the tongue is dry with cracking or fissure formation; the tongue coating will be white, yellow or black.

2. Yin Deficiency

The tongue is deep, dull red color. It usually occurs in chronic diseases and in the latter stages of febrile disease. The patient reports sensations of flushing of the face and internal heat in the afternoon. The tongue coating is scanty or there is none at all; the surface of the tongue is dry. The patient wants to drink water. The pulse is rapid and thin.

Any localized redness on the tongue proper corresponds to the accumulation of Heat in a specific organ:

Location:	Corresponding Organ:
the center of tongue	Spleen and Stomach
the root of tongue	Kidney
the tip of tongue	Heart
the border of tongue	Liver

C. Purplish Tongue Proper

1. Interior Retention of pathogenic Heat

The tongue proper is a purple color with tones of deep red. The coating of the tongue is dry, yellow, and the surface is cracked. There may be large purplish red spots on the surface of the tongue. This kind of the tongue proper usually develops from the deep red tongue proper as the pathogenic Heat causes the stagnation of Blood.

2.   Pathogenic Cold

The tongue proper is light purple with a greenish hue. This kind of tongue proper develops from the pale tongue and it indicates that an accumulation of pathogenic Cold has caused the stagnation of Blood. The tongue has no coating, but it is moist and slippery. The size of the tongue is usually smaller than normal. This color of the tongue proper usually occurs in Deficient syndromes of the Liver and Kidneys in which pathogenic Cold has directly attacked these two organs.

3.   Stasis of Blood

The tongue proper is dark purple and there is moisture on the surface of the tongue. Dark purplish spots can be seen on the border or tip of the tongue.

THE DIFFERENTIAL DIAGNOSIS OF TONGUE COATING

A. White Tongue Coating

The white tongue coating is associated with the lung and it dominates Exterior syndromes and Cold syndromes. The tongue proper that accompanies a white coating is usually pale, though it may be slightly red and occasionally it will appear as deep red or purple .

1.   Exterior Cold

The white tongue coating often occurs at the onset of an Exogenous Wind-Cold syndrome. The tongue proper is slightly red or pale with a thin, white tongue coating that is moist. The patient will be intolerant of the cold.

2.   Exterior Heat

At the onset of a febrile disease, the tongue proper may be bright red with a thin, dry, white tongue coating. The patient will be intolerant of the cold.

3.   Interior Retention of Damp Cold

The tongue coating is white, thick and sticky. The surface of the tongue is moist and slippery.

4.   Excessive Heat

The tongue coating is white and dry and there will be cracks in the surface. The granular coating is clear. The pathogenic heat has been transmitted from the exterior to the interior of the body. This kind of tongue coating usually occurs in the middle stage of a febrile disease or in a Damp-Heat syndrome.

B. Yellow Tongue Coating

The yellow tongue coating reflects the condition of the stomach and it dominates the syndrome of Interior Heat. The tongue proper is red or deep red.

1.   Exterior Heat Invades the Interior

The tongue has a yellow coating that is thin, or slight thick, and moist with a clear, granular texture. The border of the tongue is slight red. The tip of the tongue has a white coating and the yellow coating is at the root of the tongue. This indicates that Exterior Heat has moved to the interior part of the body, or, that the pathogenic Cold has developed into Fire.

2.   Excessive Heat in the Stomach

The tongue coating is a deep yellow color and it is dry and sticky. Occasionally, the papillary buds are visibly red and there will be cracking in the surface of the tongue associated with a gray or black color. The pathogenic Heat has invaded the stomach.

3.   Damp-Heat

The tongue coating is yellow, sticky, slippery and moist. The patient will have yellow urine and the the sclera of the eyes will appear to be slightly yellow.

C. Grayish-Black Tongue Coating

A grayish-black tongue coating occurs in the last stages of prolonged disease. The endogenous Cold or Cold-Damp has accumulated in the interior of the body due to Yang Deficiency.

1.   Exhausted Yin due to extreme Heat

The tongue proper is pale and the surface of the tongue is covered with a thin, moist grayish-black coating. The tongue coating has changed from yellow to grayish black. This occurs in prolonged febrile diseases in which the excessive pathogenic Heat has been transmitted to interior of the body and has exhausted the Yin.

2.   Endogenous Cold due to Yang Deficiency

The tongue proper is pale and the coating is a thin, moist, and grayish-black in color.

3.   Kidney Deficiency

The tongue is small with a dry, grayish-black tongue coating. The patient has symptoms of Deficiency of the Kidney, but there are no Heat signs. This is a Yin Deficiency due to Deficiency of the essential fluid of the Kidney.

Chapter IV

The Eight Principles

CHAPTER IV. THE EIGHT PRINCIPLES

The concept of the Eight Principles in Chinese medicine involves the following sets of complimentary opposites:

YIN and YANG	XU and SHI
INTERIOR and EXTERIOR	COLD and HEAT

All diseases are either Yin or Yang in nature. All syndromes of Shi (excess), Exterior and Heat are Yang. All syndromes of Xu (deficiency), Interior and Cold are Yin. The Principle of Xu and Shi refers to the relative strength or weakness of the body in resisting a pathogenic factor in the progress of disease. Interior and Exterior refers to the depth to which the disease has entered the body. Finally, Cold and Heat refers to the nature of the disease.

YIN AND YANG

A. The clinical signs of a Yang syndrome

   a. anxiety
   b. preference for brightness or light
   c. coarse or rough respiration
   d. preference for cold
   e. thirsty and likes to drink water
   f. yellow urine
   g. constipation
   h. warm hands and feet
   i. fever
   j. superficial and rapid pulse

B. The clinical signs of a Yin syndrome

   a. dislikes speaking
   b. dislikes brightness or light
   c. weak respiration
   d. responds well to warmth
   e. intolerance of cold
   f. clear urine
   g. bowel movement is without a bad smell

    h.   cold hands and feet
    i.   deep and slow pulse

C. Insufficiency of True Yin (Jen Yin) and True Yang (Jen Yang)

The two syndromes of Insufficiency of True Yin and of True Yang are due to deficiencies of the Yin Qi and the Yang Qi. Both Yin and Yang deficiencies belong to (are associated with) the Kidneys. Thus, Insufficiency of True Yin means that the Yin, or Water, of the Kidneys is deficient. The pulse associated with Kidney Yin, or the Water of the Kidney, is the pulse of the Chi region of the right hand. In this case, it will be weak. Similarly, Insufficiency of True Yang means that the Yang, or Fire, of the Kidneys is deficient. Kidney Yang is associated with the pulse at the Chi region of the left hand and it will be thin and rapid.

    1.   Insufficiency of True Yin

This syndrome involves the upward rising of deficient fire and is associated with dryness of the mouth and tongue, feverish feelings and constipation. The pulse is rapid and forceless.

    2.   Insufficiency of True Yang

The signs and symptoms of this syndrome include cold in the four limbs, soft or watery stool, indigestion, pale lips, fatigue, and a pulse that is wide and weak.

D. Collapse of Yin and Collapse of Yang

In the advanced stages of disease, the severe syndromes of collapse of the Yin and the Yang occur. The signs and symptoms associated with these syndromes are very high fever, excessive sweating, excessive vomiting or diarrhea, and excessive hemorrhage.

    1.   The Clinical Signs of Syndrome of Collapse of Yin

        a.   excessive and sticky sweating
        b.   thirsty and likes to drink cold water
        c.   the skin (body surface) is hot and both the hands and feet are warm

       d.   flushed face and ears
       e.   shallow and rapid breathing
       f.   exhaustion
       g.   wide and rapid pulse

2.   The Clinical Signs of Syndrome of Collapse of Yang

       a.   pallor
       b.   no thirst but desire to drink hot water
       c.   the skin (body surface) is cold as are both the hands
           and feet
       d.   intolerance of cold
       e.   feeble respiration
       f.   exhaustion
       g.   feeble and rapid pulse

EXTERIOR AND INTERIOR

A syndrome that is presenting as Cold or as Heat, as Xu (deficiency) or as Shi (excess) can manifest as an Exterior or as an Interior syndrome.

A. Clinical Manifestations of Exterior Syndromes

1.   Exterior Cold

       a.   headache
       b.   neck stiffness
       c.   chills
       d.   no sweat
       e.   achiness in the joints
       f.   thin, white tongue coating
       g.   superficial and forceful pulse

2.   Exterior Heat

       a.   fever
       b.   slight intolerance to wind
       c.   sweating or absence of sweating
       d.   thirst
       e.   superficial and rapid pulse

3. Exterior Xu (deficiency)

   a. fever
   b. intolerance to wind
   c. sweating
   d. superficial and slow pulse

4. Exterior Shi (excess)

   a. fever
   b. intolerance to cold
   c. no sweat
   d. superficial and forceful pulse

B. Clinical manifestations of Interior Syndromes

1. Interior Cold

   a. no sweat
   b. cold in the four limbs
   c. nausea and vomiting
   d. diarrhea and abdominal pain
   e. white and moist tongue coating
   f. deep and slow pulse

2. Interior Heat

   a. high fever
   b. intolerance to heat
   c. thirsty and likes to drink cold water
   d. emotional state is anxious and upset
   e. flushed face
   f. red tongue with yellow coating
   g. wide and rapid pulse

3. Interior Xu (deficiency)

   a. loss of appetite
   b. cold in the four limbs
   c. palpitations
   d. dizziness

    e. general weakness
    f. flabby and pale tongue proper with a thin white coating

4. Interior Shi (excess)

    a. sweating in both the hands and feet
    b. fever
    c. chest fullness
    d. constipation
    e. abdominal distension
    f. coarse respiration
    g. rough tongue proper with thick yellow coating
    h. deep and forceful pulse

C. Clinical Manifestations of both Exterior and Interior Simultaneously

It is possible for different conditions to be present at the same time. These syndromes reveal combinations of symptoms and manifest on different levels in the course of a disease.

1. Exterior Cold with Interior Heat

This condition begins with Exterior Cold that is not eliminated and develops into Interior Heat. The symptoms are:

    a. fever
    b. intolerance to cold
    c. the whole body is painful
    d. absence of sweating
    e. anxiety
    f. superficial and forceful pulse

2. Exterior Heat with Interior Cold

    a. headache with fever
    b. slight intolerance to wind and cold
    c. diarrhea
    d. deep pulse

3. Exterior Excess with Interior Deficiency

The Interior Qi is deficient and an external pathogenic factor causes an Exterior Excess condition.

    a. the whole body is painful
    b. diarrhea
    c. stagnation of Qi
    d. abdominal pain and distension
    e. deep and slow pulse

4. Exterior Deficiency with Interior Excess

    a. Yang deficiency
    b. indigestion
    c. phlegm accumulation
    d. sweating
    e. intolerance to wind
    f. abdominal distension
    g. difficulty in moving bowels

5. Both Exterior and Interior Cold

    a. no sweating
    b. the whole body is cold
    c. watery stool
    d. thin, deep and slow pulse

6. Both Exterior and Interior Heat

    a. panting and sweating
    b. diarrhea
    c. rapid pulse

7. Both Exterior and Interior Deficiency

    a. sweating
    b. the feeling of being cold
    c. general weakness
    d. thin and weak pulse

8. Both Exterior and Interior Excess

    a. indigestion
    b. constipation
    c. heat and water retention
    d. wide, rapid and forceful pulse

D. Clinical Manifestations of Semi-Exterior and Semi-Interior

In this case, the pathogenic factor is neither on the exterior nor the interior of the body. It is a complicated syndrome resulting in the symptoms of:

    a. intermittent feelings of cold and heat
    b. pain in the lateral aspect of the chest
    c. anxiety and nausea
    d. lack of appetite
    e. a bitter taste in the mouth
    f. dryness in the pharynx
    g. dizziness
    h. white and greasy tongue coating
    i. wiry and thin pulse

In the course of the development of disease, an Exterior syndrome may move to the Interior and an Interior syndrome move to the Exterior. The former marks the worsening of the disease while the latter indicates recovery from a severe condition.

E. Exterior Syndrome Moving to the Interior

If the patient has clear, copious urine, the pathogenic factor has not moved into the Interior. There are two specific conditions that indicate an interior movement in the disease process.

1. The patient has symptoms of nausea and vomiting, bitter taste in the mouth, chest fullness and lack of appetite. The exogenous pathogenic factor is affecting the chest and the internal organs.

2. The patient has symptoms of anxiety, insomnia, abdominal distension, and lack of control of urination. The pathogen

has attacked the internal organs.

F. Interior Syndrome Moving to Exterior

The interior symptoms of anxiety, chest fullness and nausea become the symptoms of fever with sweating and a rash.

COLD AND HEAT

A. The Clinical Signs of Cold Syndrome

    a.   absence of thirst or thirst without desire to drink fluids
    b.   hands and feet are cold
    c.   pale complexion
    d.   clear urine with increased volume
    e.   diarrhea with watery stool
    f.   white and slippery tongue coating
    g.   slow pulse

B. The Clinical Signs of Heat Syndrome

    a.   thirst with desire to drink cold water
    b.   flushed face
    c.   constipation
    d.   concentrated urine
    e.   anxiety
    f.   yellow tongue coating that is rough
    g.   rapid pulse

C. Cold and Heat Syndromes in the Upper or Lower Part of the Body

    1.   Cold Syndrome in the Upper Part of the Body

        a.   indigestion
        b.   retention of food in the throat
        c.   abdominal distention
        d.   nausea and hiccough

2. Cold Syndrome in the Lower Part of the Body

    a. diarrhea
    b. abdominal pain
    c. hernia
    d. hands and feet are cold

3. Heat Syndrome in the Upper Part of the Body

    a. headache
    b. redness of the eyes
    c. sore throat
    d. toothache

4. Heat Syndrome in the Lower Part of the Body

    a. the lumbar area of the back and the feet are swollen and painful
    b. constipation
    c. concentrated yellow urine

D. The Syndromes of True and False Cold/Heat

There exists a phenomenon that occurs when Heat syndromes develop to the extreme outcome and present symptoms of Cold and vice versa.

1. True Heat with False Cold

Extreme Heat accumulates on the interior of the body and causes stagnation of the Yang Qi. The Yang Qi can not spread over the exterior part of the body and the symptoms that appear seem to suggest signs of Cold.

    a. cold in the four limbs
    b. coarse respiration
    c. dryness in the pharynx
    d. abdominal distention and pain
    e. constipation
    f. concentrated urine
    g. heat retention in the urinary bladder

     h.   tongue coating is yellowish/black color
     i.   pulse is deep and forceful

2. True Cold with False Heat

Excess Yin Cold causes the Yang Qi to go to the exterior parts of the body adding signs of Heat to a Cold syndrome.

     a.   cold sweating
     b.   extreme cold in hands and feet
     c.   feeble voice
     d.   dryness in the mouth and pain in the pharynx
     e.   clear urine
     f.   anxiety
     g.   thirst but drinks only small amounts of fluid
     h.   tongue proper is flabby and soft with a grayish-black coating in the center
     i.   thin and weak pulse

XU (DEFICIENCY) and SHI (EXCESS)

A. The general symptoms of a Deficient syndrome

     a.   a chronic disorder or prolonged illness
     b.   pallor
     c.   feeble respiration and shortness of breath
     d.   night sweating
     e.   bowel movement that is soft and loose
     f.   clear urine with increased volume
     g.   vomiting
     h.   blurred vision
     i.   pale tongue proper with thin coating
     j.   thin, weak pulse

B. The general symptoms of an Excessive syndrome

     a.   recent disease with a strong body constitution
     b.   exhaustion
     c.   chest fullness
     d.   abdominal distention
     e.   constipation

  f. difficult urination
  g. coarse respiration
  h. red tongue proper with thick coating

C. Syndromes of Deficiency and Excess of Qi/Blood

Deficiency of Qi   Excess of Qi

a. shortness of breath   a. Phlegm-Heat
b. apathy   b. Damp-Heat
c. indigestion   c. indigestion
d. palpitations   d. chest fullness
e. anxiety   e. abdominal distention
f. dizziness   f. constipation
g. tinnitus   g. diarrhea
h. sweating
i. general lassitude
j. feeble pulse

Deficiency of Blood

a. anxiety
b. insomnia
c. night sweating
d. dryness of skin
e. pale lips
f. thin and forceless pulse

Excess of Blood

The concept of Excess of Blood implies blood stagnation and the signs and symptoms depend on where the blood stagnation is located.

Location of Blood Stasis:	Clinical Manifestations:
internal organs	intermittent cold and heat symptoms
muscles	fever and sweating
Jing Luo (meridians)	pain in the muscles and tendons

upper jiao (chest region)	pain in the hypochondriac region; forgetfulness; purple tongue coating
middle jiao (upper abdominal area)	abdominal pain; stomach ache; black stool
lower jiao (lower abdominal area)	abdominal distention; frequent urination

D. The Syndromes of True and False Deficiency/Excess

In a condition of severe Deficiency where extreme Cold is transformed into Heat, signs of an Excessive syndrome can appear. This is known as a "pseudo-phenomenon" syndrome.

If a disorder results from an imbalance of the seven emotional factors and if it is chronic, there may appear together signs and symptoms of both deficiency and excess, such as constipation, chest fullness and heat in the body.

In a condition of severe Excess where extreme Heat is transformed into Cold, the syndrome is also referred to as a "pseudo-phenomenon" syndrome, that of True Excess/False Deficiency. If a disorder results from a pathogenic factor that is not completely eliminated and stays in the Jing Luo (meridians), there will be some signs of deficiency such as indigestion, stagnation of Qi and Blood, and fatigue along with signs of an Excessive syndrome.

Chapter V

Differential Diagnosis According to

the Function of

Qi and Xue (Blood)

CHAPTER V: DIFFERENTIAL DIAGNOSIS ACCORDING TO THE FUNCTION OF QI AND XUE (BLOOD)

SYNDROMES OF THE QI

Pathological changes in the Qi are categorized as Qi Deficiency and Qi Stagnation.

A. Qi Deficiency

The symptoms of Qi Deficiency are:

     a.   fatigue
     b.   the voice is weak and low
     c.   shortness of breath
     d.   spontaneous sweating
     e.   pale or flabby tongue proper
     f.   thin and forceless pulse

Deficiency of the Qi of the internal organs is related to the physiological function of each organ.

Organ:	Function:	Symptoms:
Lung	dominating the Qi	shortness of breath no desire to speak low voice cough with sputum
Heart	controlling the blood vessels and housing the mind	shortness of breath fatigue palpitations anxiety intermittent, short, slow or rapid pulse

Spleen and Stomach	governing transportation and transformation of alimentary nutrients	pale face fatigue loss of appetite abdominal distention indigestion watery stool frequent urination
Kidney	storing essential substance; producing marrow and receiving Qi	pale face dizziness ringing in the ears weakness in the lumbar area and knees clear urine incontinence of urine or retention of urine impotence

Qi is considered to be Yang in nature. The characteristics of Qi Deficiency and Yang Deficiency are similar. The fundamental clinical sign that distinguishes one syndrome from the other is the degree to which Cold predominates. In Qi Deficiency, the "Cold phenomenon" is not prominent whereas in Yang Deficiency, the "Cold phenomenon" is prominent. For example, if a patient has a syndrome of Qi Deficiency with a Cold phenomenon presenting as cold in the hands and feet, intolerance to cold, cold sweating and a slow pulse, it is a syndrome of Yang Deficiency.

B. Qi Stagnation

Qi Stagnation is usually the result of imbalances in the diet, the emotions, or the life style of the patient. Exogenous pathogenic factors can also be the cause of Qi Stagnation. The main clinical sign of Stagnation of Qi is pain and distention. The pain usually moves from one site to another (" wandering pain") rather than being fixed and is often related to an emotional factor.

1.   Stagnation of Qi in the chest causes chest pain and fullness

2.   Stagnation of Qi in the gastrointestinal tract causes pain and distention in the stomach and abdomen

3. Stagnation of Qi in the joints causes pain and stiffness in the joints

4. Stagnation of Qi in the Liver meridian causes pain in the breast area

The syndrome of Qi Stagnation is associated with mental and emotional disorders, physical trauma, and functional gastrointestinal disorders such as chronic gastritis, chronic enteritis, ulcerative disorders, gall bladder disorders and chronic hepatitis.

SYNDROMES OF THE XUE (BLOOD)

There are three major categories of syndromes which affect the Blood: Deficiency of Blood; Stasis of Blood; and Heat in the Blood. These three syndromes have an interdependent relationship with hemorrhage in that Deficiency of Blood and the Stasis of Blood may result from hemorrhage and vice versa.

A. Blood Deficiency

The symptoms of Blood Deficiency are:

a. pallor
b. dizziness
c. diminished vision
d. pale tongue proper
e. thin pulse

The syndrome of Blood Deficiency can arise from a number of factors:

1. blood loss without adequate production of blood to replenish supply
2. the Spleen and Stomach fails in the function of transportation and transformation of nutritive Qi
3. prolonged hematoma
4. dysfunction of the hematopoietic organs.

The theory of the Zang-Fu of Chinese medical science indicates that the heart controls the blood, the liver stores the blood and the spleen contains and manufactures blood. Thus, Blood Deficiency is greatly related to the physiological function of the heart, spleen and liver.

Blood is Yin in nature. The syndromes of Blood Deficiency and Yin Deficiency have similar characteristics with one important exception: Blood Deficiency has no "heat phenomenon". Yin Deficiency has a prominent phenomena of dryness and heat that is known as "Empty Fire". It is due to an insufficiency of body fluid. The symptoms include a flushed face, a feeling of internal heat or the hyperactivity of the Yang Qi, a thin and rapid pulse, and a red tongue proper.

Specific clinical manifestations will be present when Deficient Blood affects a particular organ:

Organ:	Symptoms:
Heart	palpitations
	forgetfulness (amnesia)
	vivid dreams
	insomnia
Both Heart and Spleen	symptoms of Blood Deficiency plus: loss of appetite
	fatigue
	irregular menstruation
	anemia
Liver	symptoms of Blood Deficiency plus: numbness in the hands and feet
	anxiety
	muscle and joint stiffness
	poor sleep
	irregular or scanty menstruation
	amenorrhea

B. Stasis of the Blood

The symptoms of Stasis of the Blood are:

a. pain

Pain that is sharp and fixed in a specific location is the

most common clinical sign of stasis of the Blood. The blood vessels and meridians are obstructed by the Stasis of blood.

b. hematoma

A hematoma is a subcutaneous bruise that is blue and purple in color and results from physical injury; it may also be a hard mass of tissue that results from deep tissue damage or damaged internal organs.

c. hemorrhage

Hemorrhage often occurs post-partum or with irregular menstruation. The blood is deep purple in color and there may be clots.

d. systemic symptoms

In cases where there is chronic Stasis of Blood, there will be symptoms of dry skin, red or purple spots on the skin, grayish-black color on the face and around the eyes, a greenish tendon prominently showing on the abdominal area, a deep purple tongue proper with or without purple spots.

Stasis of the Blood usually results from the syndromes of Qi Stagnation, Qi Deficiency, Cold Blood, and Heat in the Blood. Common conditions that are related to Blood Stagnation are the various post-hemorrhages, sports injuries and other physical injuries, cardiovascular disorders, CVA (cerebro-vascular accident), hepatosplenomegaly, menstrual disorders, and post-partum disorders.

C. Heat in the Blood

The symptoms of Heat in the Blood are:

a. anxiety
b. thirst
c. a deep red tongue proper

d. a rapid pulse
e. coma (if severe)

The syndrome of Heat in the Blood is associated with an increase in blood volume that is either a fresh red or a dark purple color and a red rash on the skin.

Heat in the Blood usually occurs with exogenous febrile diseases. It also is present with internal disorders such as leukemia, aplastic anemia, urticaria, allergic purpura, and thrombopenic purpura. Heat in the Blood injures the blood vessels and meridians causes abnormal bleeding of the affected parts, for example, blood in the urine or stool, epistaxis, hemoptysis, and polymenorrhea.

SYNDROMES INVOLVING BOTH QI AND BLOOD

Qi and Blood are closely related in terms of both physiology and pathology. The clinical manifestations of the syndromes of the Qi and the Blood often show signs and symptoms of both.

A. Stagnation of Qi and Stasis of Blood

The two separate syndromes of Stagnation of Qi and Stasis of Blood often occur together. Among the conditions that arise from this combination are irregular menstruation, clotted blood in the menstruation, abdominal pain associated with menstruation, breast pain and distention, chronic hepatitis, ulcerative disorders, and physical injury. The treatment for these conditions is to regulate Qi and activate the Blood.

B. Deficiency of both Qi and Blood

The syndromes of Qi Deficiency and Blood Deficiency can occur together and are often found in cases such as anemia and hemorrhagic disorders. Chinese medical science states that "Blood is the mother of the Qi". The patient with Blood Deficiency will usually have a syndrome of Qi Deficiency as well showing typical symptoms such as shortness of breath and fatigue. The treatment for the syndromes of Deficiency of both Qi and Blood is to tonify both the Qi and the Blood. In general, this approach to treatment emphasizes the tonification of the Qi since this will strengthen blood circulation and enhance the function of the hematapoietic organs (liver, spleen, etc.).

Chapter VI

Differential diagnosis According to the

Theory of Zang-Fu (Internal Organs)

CHAPTER VI. DIFFERENTIAL DIAGNOSIS ACCORDING TO THE THEORY OF ZANG-FU (INTERNAL ORGANS)

In order to diagnose a condition according to the theory of the Zang-Fu, it is essential to understand the syndromes that affect the internal organs and the pathological changes as they relate to Yin, Yang, Qi and Blood.

CONCEPTS

A. The Physiology and Pathology of the Internal Organs

1. Heart

The heart has the function of controlling the blood vessels and of housing the mind. The symptoms of pathology in the functioning of the heart are palpitations, mental confusion, and a knotted and intermittent pulse.

2. Lung

The lung has the function of governing the Qi in dispersing it and causing it to descend properly, controlling respiration, and dominating the skin and the hair. The pathological manifestations of the lung include cough, asthma, and susceptibility to colds.

3. Spleen, Stomach and Intestine

The spleen governs the transportation and transformation of Qi; the stomach receives food and begins digestion; the intestines continue with the digestive process, absorbing essential substances and water from food (in the small intestine) and turning fluid content into feces (in the large intestine). Indigestion, abdominal distention and diarrhea are common pathological manifestations of the spleen, stomach and intestine.

4. Liver

The liver is responsible for maintaining the potency of the flow of Qi, storing the blood, and for governing the tendons. The Yang of the

Liver tends to move in an upward direction. This produces the symptoms of pain in the hypochondriac region, jaundice, dimness of sight, hemorrhage, and muscle spasm.

5. Kidney

The function of the Kidney is to govern the stages of growth and development; the Kidney is said to "dominate reproduction". The Kidney also receives Qi, produces marrow and dominates the bones, regulates fluid, and stores essential substances.

Among the pathological symptoms of Kidney syndromes are edema, retention of urine, incontinence of urine, seminal emission, weakness and soreness of the lumbar area and the knees, and slow movement.

B. The Relationship Between The Internal Organs and Pathological Changes

Organ:	Energetic Changes:
Lung	Qi; Yin
Heart	Yin; Yang; Qi; Blood
Spleen	Qi; Yang
Kidney	Yin; Yang; Essential Qi
Liver	Yin; Yang; Qi; Blood

If, for example, a patient has heart palpitations, the syndrome will involve the Heart. It must be determined whether there is Deficient Yin of the Heart, Deficient Yang of the Heart, Deficient Qi of the Heart or Deficient Blood of the Heart.

The internal organs are functionally interrelated. The effects of a disease process on one organ system must be assessed in terms of the effects on the other related organs. For example, in the treatment of insomnia, there will be Blood Deficiency of the Heart or Deficiency of Yin of the Heart; but there may be pathological changes affecting the Spleen or the Kidney. If the Kidney is affected, the differential diagnosis will be disharmony of the Heart and Kidney. If the Spleen is affected, the differential diagnosis will be Deficiency of Blood of both Heart and Spleen.

SYNDROMES OF THE ZANG-FU (INTERNAL ORGANS)

A. The Heart

1. Deficient Heart Qi and Deficient Heart Yang

Though these are two different kinds of diseases, both of them are the result of a prolonged disorder. They usually occur in conditions such as heart failure, cardialgia, cardi-asthma, general weakness, and nervous system dysfunction.

Syndrome:	Signs and Symptoms:
Deficient Heart Qi	pallor; fatigue; poor eyesight; palpitation; shortness of breath; spontaneous sweating; pale tongue proper; slow, thin and weak pulse that may sometimes be knotted and intermittent
Deficient Heart Yang	Deficient Heart Qi symptoms plus: cold in the four limbs; stasis of the blood
Extreme Heart Yang Deficiency	excessive sweating; edema in the face and feet; dizziness; thin and weak pulse

2. Deficient Heart Blood and Deficient Heart Yin

Deficiency of the Blood of the Heart and Deficiency of the Yin of the Heart result from a chronic disorder whereby the Yin of the Blood is exhausted. These conditions are associated with emotional or mental illnesses. Both of them usually occur in conditions such as general malnutrition, tachycardia, anemia, and hyperthyroidism.

The major clinical signs of Deficient Heart Blood and Deficient Heart Yin are anxiety and insufficiency of the Blood Yin.

Syndrome: Signs and Symptoms:

Deficient   pale face; palpitations; poor vision;
Heart Blood   forgetfulness; insomnia; anxiety; dream-
                             disturbed sleep; pale tongue proper and thin
                             pulse

Deficient   palpitations; poor vision; insomnia;
Heart Yin   dream-disturbed sleep; anxiety; night
                             sweating; red tongue proper; chest fullness;
                             thin and rapid pulse

3. Hyperactivity of Heart Fire

This belongs to the Shi syndrome (excessive syndrome). If it is associated with hyperactivity of the fire of the liver, it will be called hyperactivity of the fire of both heart and liver, and sometimes the heat
can be transferred to small intestine and cause indigestions. If it is
associated with deficiency of the Yin of the kidney, it will be called
disharmony of the Qi of heart and kidney, which belongs to syndrome
of hyperactivity of the fire of the Yin deficiency.

Syndrome: Signs and Symptoms:

Hyperactivity of   anxiety; red tongue tip; rapid pulse
Heart Fire

Fire of both the   headache; red eyes; anxiety; if the Fire
Heart and   invades the small intestine; the patient
the Liver   will have painful urination

Disharmony of the   anxiety; dryness in pharynx; flushed
Qi of both the Heart   face; red tongue proper; thin and
the Kidney   rapid pulse

4. Stasis of Heart Blood

This condition results from insufficient Yang Qi, poor circulation, stagnation of the Qi in the meridians due to sticky phlegm, and obstructed
blood vessels in the heart due to stasis of the Blood. Stasis of the Blood
of the Heart is associated with myocardial obstruction and cardialgia.

Syndrome:	Signs and Symptoms:
Stasis of Heart Blood	palpitations; pain and fullness in the left side of the chest; shortness of breath; cold in the four limbs; cyanosis of lips and nails; dark purplish tongue proper or purple spots on the tongue; thin and weak pulse or missed beats

B. The Lung

The major physiological functions of the Lung are that of dispersing and descending the Qi. The symptoms of coughing and shallow, rapid respiration are characteristic of a Lung disharmony.

   1.   Dysfunction of the Ability of the Lung to Disperse the Qi

Whenever exogenous factors invade the Lung or restrain the surface of the body, the dispersing function of the Lung is diminished.

Syndrome:	Signs and Symptoms:
Dysfunction of the dispersing of the Qi of the Lung	cough; fever; panting with coarse breath; sticky yellowish phlegm (may contain a little blood); deep red tongue proper with yellow coating; rolling (slippery) and rapid pulse

   2.   Dysfunction of the Ability of the Lung to Descend the Qi

The Lung will loose its ability to descend the Qi when the invasion of exogenous factors develops into Heat causing the interior retention of Damp-Phlegm in the lung.

The major symptom of the Qi failing to descend properly is a persistent cough. The symptoms associated with a persistent cough will differ depending on whether the Heat has changed into Damp-Heat.

Syndrome:	Signs and Symptoms:
Pathogenic Heat or Dryness	dry cough with little or no sputum; dry pharynx and difficult speech

If the patient suffers from tuberculosis and has this kind of cough, the syndrome will develop into deficiency of Lung Yin.

Interior Retention of Damp-Phlegm	cough; sticky phlegm; chest fullness sticky tongue coating; rolling (slippery) pulse.

In severe cases, the patient may have asthma or chronic bronchitis and the condition can easily develop into Deficient Lung Qi.

3. Deficient Lung Qi

Deficient Lung Qi results from the prolonged inability of the Lung to descend or disperse the Qi. It may have an adverse effect on the function of the Lung in transporting essential Qi to the skin and hair. This, in turn, weakens the Wei Qi (Defensive Qi) in its role of protecting against exogenous factors.

The Qi of the Lung is connected to the Kidney; the Zhong Qi (Essential Qi) nourishes the Heart and assists in respiration. Chronic Deficiency of Lung Qi will develop into Deficiency of the Qi of both the Lung and the Heart, dysfunction of the Kidney in receiving the Qi and Deficiency of Yang of both the Heart and the Kidney.

The clinical manifestations of Deficient Lung Qi include:

- a. general weakness
- b. fatigue
- c. the voice is low and weak
- d. cough
- e. shortness of breath
- f. pale tongue proper
- g. weak pulse

Syndrome:	Symptoms:
Deficient Lung Qi injures the Wei Qi (Defensive Qi)	spontaneous sweating; nasal obstruction; common cold

Deficient Lung Qi injures the Yang Qi	panting; pronounced cold in the four limbs; edema of the face and feet
Extremely weakened Yang Qi of Heart or Kidney	chest fullness with shortness of breath; palpitations; spontaneous sweating; purple color of the lips

4. Deficient Lung Yin

Deficient Lung Yin develops from prolonged illness with the dysfunction of the descending of the Qi of the Lung and prolonged stagnation of pathogenic Heat in the Lung.

Deficient Lung Yin is a pattern of Lung Deficiency with a "heat phenomenon". It occurs in the condition of pulmonary tuberculosis or occasionally if pathogenic Dryness invades the Lung. Deficient Lung Yin often injures the Kidney Yin resulting in Yin Deficiency of both the Lung and the Kidney.

Syndrome:	Symptoms:
Deficient Lung Yin	dry mouth and throat with scanty saliva; lower voice; sputum may contain blood; panting; flushed face; the feeling of internal heat; slight afternoon fever; night sweating; general debility; soreness in the lumbar area,; nocturnal emission; red tongue proper; thin and rapid pulse
Deficient Lung and Kidney Yin	dizziness; mild headache; night sweating; feverish sensation in palms and soles of the feet; thready and rapid pulse

C. The Liver

The Liver functions in storing the blood, regulating the flow of Qi and controlling the tendons. The syndromes of Liver disorders stem from an excess of Liver Qi or Liver Yang, and a deficiency of Liver Yin or Liver Blood.

1. Depression of Liver Qi (Constrained Liver Qi)

Depression of Liver Qi results from a number of imbalances and disorders including irregular menses and pre-menstrual syndrome (specifically breast swelling), mental and emotional irritation, poor gastrointestinal function, ulcerative disorders, chronic hepatitis and hepatic cirrhosis. The syndromes associated with Depression of Liver Qi are exogenous Damp Heat and Deficient Liver Yin.

The clinical signs and symptoms of Depression of Liver Qi vary according to the following factors:

Etiological Factor:	Symptoms:
mental and emotional factors	depression; anxiety
Liver Qi disharmony	fullness, swelling and/or pain in the hypochondriac region; chest fullness; wiry pulse
Gallbladder dysfunction with bile secretion	vomiting with bitter water; nausea
Liver Qi invades the Stomach	nausea,; vomiting; abdominal pain
Disharmony of the Liver Qi and the Spleen Qi	diarrhea; abdominal pain
Chong Mai and Ren Mai injured by stasis of Liver Qi	menorrhalgia; breast swelling and pain during menstruation; irregular menstruation

2.   Liver Fire Ascending

Liver Fire Ascending is a Shi (excess) syndrome that develops from prolonged stagnation of Liver Qi, severe mental irritation or interior retention of pathogenic Damp-Heat. In this condition, the Fire of the Liver flares upwards to the head and facial area. This is known as a "heat phenomenon". Liver fire Ascending often adversely affects the function of Liver in storing the Blood and can result in abnormal bleeding or hemorrhage.

Syndrome: Symptoms:

Liver Fire Ascending   tension headache; flushed face; red eyes;
                       ringing in both ears or sudden deafness;
                       vomiting of bitter or acidic fluid; dry stool
                       or constipation; anxiety; anger dominates
                       emotions; red tongue proper with thick,
                       rough, yellow coating; wiry and slippery
                       pulse

When Liver Fire Ascending impairs the Liver in its function of storing the Blood, the symptoms of hematemesis, epistaxis and profuse
menstruation can occur.

   3. Liver Yang Ascending

The disharmony of Liver Yin and Liver Yang due to Yin Deficiency
of both the Liver and the Kidney results in Liver Yang Ascending.
This configuration occurs in such conditions as acute hepatitis, acute
kidney disorders such as nephritis, acute or chronic gall bladder in-
flammation, hepatonephromegaly, and hepatoperitonitis.

Syndrome: Symptoms:

Liver Yang Ascending   headache and head distention; anger
                       dominates emotions; flushed face; red eyes;
                       ringing in the ears; insomnia; weakness in
                       the legs; red tongue proper; wiry and thin
                       pulse

The differential diagnosis of Depression of Liver Qi, Liver Yang Ascending, and Liver Fire Ascending are briefly described as follows:

   a. Depression of Liver Qi is due to the inability of the Liver
       to disperse the Liver Qi. The Yin of the Liver is injured
       allowing the Yang of the Liver to move upward.

   b. The disturbance of Liver Yang and its movement upward to
       the head and face results from Deficient Liver Yin. The
       Yin of the Liver can not control the Yang of the Liver.

c. Liver Fire Ascending develops from the stagnation and depression of the Qi of the Liver which transforms into the Fire and moves upward.

4. Liver Wind Stirred Up by Heat

The Wind of the Liver is an endogenous (internal) Wind that is Xu (Deficient)in nature. It arises from excessive impairment of the Yin of the Liver and the Kidney which are in turn unable to nourish the Yang of the Liver. The Yang of the Liver is transformed into Wind. Liver Wind is the final development of the Liver syndromes of Deficient Yin and Blood of the Liver, Liver Yang Ascending, and Liver Fire Ascending.

Syndrome: Symptoms:

Liver Wind   severe dizziness; tension headache;
Stirred up by Heat   neck stiffness; numbness in the four limbs;
                         stiffness of the tendons; shaking of the lips,
                         tongue and fingers; difficult speech;
                         convulsion and coma in severe cases; dark
                         red tongue proper with dry coating;
                         prominent wiry pulse

5. Deficient Liver Blood

Deficient Liver Blood arises from a chronic condition whereby the Blood fails to nourish the Liver and the Liver fails to store the Blood. This occurs in such disorders as chronic hepatitis, hepatospenomegaly, hepatonecrosis, and hepatorrhagia.

Syndrome: Symptoms:

Deficient Liver Blood   fatigue; loss of weight; dizziness; diminished
                        or blurred vision; pallor; insomnia; neck
                        stiffness; loss of appetite; loss of muscle
                        strength; scanty menstruation; amenorrhea;
                        seminal emission; soreness of lumbar region;
                        infertility (if the syndromes effect the Kidney)

D. The Spleen

In Chinese medical science, the Spleen controls the Blood and governs the transportation and transformation of Qi and Blood. Pathology involving the Spleen will present as a disturbance of the digestive tract and in the absorption and transmission of fluids.

1. Dysfunction of the Ability of the Spleen to Transport Qi and Blood

The inability of the Spleen to transport Qi and Blood results from a number of factors including irregular diet, excessive mental strain, prolonged illness with general weakness and excessive mental strain or excessive hard work. The Spleen Yang is weakened and is unable to support the visceral tissues. Associated with this syndrome are Deficient Spleen Qi and invasion of the Spleen by Cold-Damp (usually due to the over-eating of cold or raw foods).

This syndrome occurs in such conditions as chronic gastritis, chronic enteritis, gastrointestinal dysfunction, chronic liver and gall bladder disorders, malnutrition, general weakness, and ptosis (dropping) of internal organs.

Syndrome:	Symptoms:
Deficient Spleen Qi	dysfunction of digestion and absorption; abdominal discomfort or pain; watery stool or diarrhea; fatigue; pale tongue proper; thin and forceless pulse
Inactivity of Spleen Yang that may injure Kidney Yang	symptoms of Deficient Spleen Qi with prominent "cold phenomenon"
Invasion of the Spleen by Cold-Damp	poor appetite; loose stools; abdominal pain; heaviness of the head; epigastric fullness and distension

2. Spleen Fails to Govern the Blood

When the Spleen Qi has become debilitated, it may fail in its function of containing the Blood in its normal vessels. Abnormal bleeding, or hemorrhage, will occur with symptoms such as uterine hemorrhage and blood in the stool.

Syndrome: Symptoms:

Spleen Fails to   symptoms of Spleen Yang Deficiency and:
Govern the Blood   pallor; fatigue; dizziness; palpitations;
                             shortness of breath; hemorrhage; pale tongue
                             proper; thin, forceless pulse

E. The Kidney

The physiological functions of the Kidney are the storing of Essential Substances; dominating human reproduction, growth and development; producing marrow; dominating body fluid; and receiving vital energy (Qi). Pathological manifestations of kidney dysfunction are deficiency of the essential substances and marrow, dysfunction of metabolism and excretion of fluids.

1.   Deficient Kidney Yin

Kidney Yin is closely related to the heart, liver and lung. Deficiency of the Yin of the Kidney is often the result of deficiencies of the heart, liver and lung. Clinical syndromes usually show Deficiency of the Yin of both the Kidney and the Heart, Deficiency of the Yin of both the Kidney and the Liver, and Deficiency of the Yin of both the Kidney and the Lung.

Syndromes: Symptoms:

Deficient Kidney   dizziness; tinnitis; dry mouth and
Yin   pharynx; interior heat sensations; soreness of
                             the lumbar area; seminal emission;
                             spontaneous sweating; red tongue proper;
                             thin and rapid pulse. In severe cases, the
                             above clinical signs are present along with
                             weight loss; fatigue; dark red tongue proper

Deficiency of both Kidney and Heart Yin	insomnia; palpitations; forgetfulness; dream-disturbed sleep. This condition occurs in tachycardia and hyperthyroidism
Deficiency of both Kidney and Liver Yin	headache; blurred vision; impaired vision; irregular menstruation; infertility. This is found in hypertension, functional disorders of the nervous system, and menstrual disorders.
Deficiency of both Kidney and Lung Yin	dry cough; sputum with blood; fever with feverish sweating. This usually occurs in pulmonary tuberculosis or chronic cough.

2. Deficient Kidney Yang

The Yang of the Kidney is closely related to the function of the spleen, lung and heart. Deficient Kidney Yang commonly results from deficiencies in the Yang of these three organs. The clinical presentation of Deficient Kidney Yang includes symptoms of Deficient Yang of the Kidney and Spleen or Deficient Yang of the Kidney and Lung.

Syndromes:	Symptoms:
Deficient Kidney Yang	dizziness; tinnitus; weakness of the lumbar area and knees; pale face; fatigue; cold in four limbs; seminal emission; impotence; polyurea or oligurea; edema; irregular menstruation; infertility; pale and flabby tongue proper; deep and thin pulse
Deficient Yang of both Kidney and Spleen	Deficient Kidney Yang signs with edema and diarrhea (especially in the morning); associated with chronic nephritis and chronic diarrhea
Deficient Yang of both Kidney and Lung	shallow, labored respiration (panting); associated with emphysema

| Deficient Yang of both Kidney and Heart | palpitations; asthma; edema; associated with heart failure |

3. Deficiency of the Essential Substances of the Kidney

Generally termed "Kidney Deficiency", this condition results from prolonged illness or congenital deficiencies.

Deficiency of the Essential Substances of the Kidney has neither a prominent "cold phenomena" nor a "heat phenomenon" as would be present in a Deficient Kidney Yang or Yin condition. It has rather a "deficient phenomenon".

Syndrome:	Symptoms:
Deficiency of the Essential Substances of the Kidney	poor intellectual development; poor bone development; impaired function of the reproductive system; hair loss; loose teeth; slow physical movement; dizziness; tinnitis; soreness of lumbar area and knees

4. Unfixation of the Qi of the Kidney

This condition reflects a debilitation of the Qi of the Kidneys. It is attributed to excessive sexual activity beginning at a young age. In the tradition of Chinese medicine, sexual behavior was to be moderate, especially in the case of early marriage. The second cause of this condition is a congenital deficiency. The clinical manifestation of this syndrome is a tendency toward cold but without a prominent "cold phenomenon".

Syndrome:	Symptoms:
Debility of the Qi of the Kidney	fatigue; weakness of the lumbar area and knees; clear urine with increased volume; incontinence of urine; impotence; seminal emission; pale tongue proper; thin and forceless pulse

F. The Stomach

The stomach and the spleen are closely related in their function of digestion and absorption. The stomach receives food from the esophagus and begins the digestive process before the food is sent downward to the small intestine. Stomach syndromes involve indicates the dysfunction of digestion and absorption.

1. Deficient-Cold Stomach Qi

Deficient-Cold Stomach Qi results from irregular food intake, the excessive intake of cold foods, or an imbalance of the emotions causing the Liver Qi to invade the stomach. This syndrome often shows in the conditions of ulceration of the stomach and nervous dysfunctional disorders of the stomach.

Syndrome:	Symptoms:
Deficient-Cold Stomach Qi	stomach ache (usually relieved after eating); vomiting with sour and cold fluid; pale face; intolerance to cold; cold sensations in the whole body; fullness and dull pain in the epigastric region; pale and flabby tongue proper; thin pulse that may become wiry and weak pulse during stomachache

Both syndromes of Deficient-Cold Stomach Qi and Invasion of Exogenous Cold will show the same symptom of stomach pain, but these syndromes can be clearly differentiated from each other. Deficient-Cold Stomach Qi has a long period of onset caused by eating too much of cold and raw foods; there will be signs of Cold and Deficiency but the Deficient Qi syndrome will be more prominent. In an exogenous Cold syndrome there will be an acute onset of symptoms with more prominent signs of a Cold syndrome.

2. Stomach Heat (Fire)

Stomach Heat is a very common Interior Heat syndrome of the internal organs. It is due to exogenous pathogenic Heat invading the stomach, eating too much food that is acrid and rich,and Liver Fire Invades the stomach. Stomach Heat is an Excess Heat syndrome and it occurs in such conditions as gastritis, ulceration of stomach, diabetes, and gingivitis.

Syndrome: Symptoms:

Stomach Heat   burning pain in the epigastric region;
                             vomiting; constipation; bitter taste in the
                             mouth; dry mouth; foul breath; gingival
                             swelling, pain or bleeding; red tongue proper
                             with rough, yellow coating ; rolling (slippery)
                             and rapid pulse

3. Deficient Stomach Yin

Deficient Stomach Yin presents during the recovery stage of exogenous Heat disorders, and after prolonged stagnation of Stomach Heat with exhaustion of stomach fluid due to prolonged illness.

Syndrome: Symptoms:

Deficient Stomach   no appetite; dry mouth; constipation;
Yin   dry vomiting; red tongue proper with no
                             coating

4. Rebellious Stomach Qi

The normal direction of the movement of the Stomach Qi is downward and when this function becomes impaired, the Qi rises upward and is referred to as Rebellious Stomach Qi. This syndrome accompanies most other stomach disorders. Rebellious Stomach Qi could arise from stomach Cold, stomach Heat, prolonged Phlegm disorder, eating contaminated food, indigestion and stagnation of the Qi of the gastrointestinal tract. The main clinical manifestations are vomiting, nausea and cough.

Syndromes: Symptoms:

Rebellious Stomach Qi   pale face; vomiting clear fluid;
due to Stomach Cold   pale tongue proper

Rebellious Stomach Qi due to Stomach Heat	vomiting with sour and bitter fluid; vomiting immediately after eating; red tongue proper with yellow coating
Rebellious Stomach Qi due to Phlegm	vomiting of saliva with little sputum; dizziness; sticky tongue coating
Rebellious Stomach Qi due to indigestion	vomiting of foul and sour undigested food; discomfort is relieved after vomiting
Rebellious Stomach Qi due to stagnation of the Qi of gastrointestinal tract	chest fullness; abdominal pain; hiccough
Rebellious Stomach Qi due to eating contaminated food	abdominal pain and distention; tendency to vomiting. This usually occurs in the summer and is an acute disorder.

G. The Intestine

The major clinical manifestations of intestinal syndromes are dysfunctions in digestion and absorption (in the small intestine) and transmission and transformation (in the large intestine).

1. Deficiency and Collapse of the Qi of the Intestine

This is caused by the collapse of the Yang Qi due to prolonged diarrhea.

Syndrome:	Symptoms:
Deficiency and Collapse of the Qi of the Intestines	persistent diarrhea; episodes of incontinence of bowel movements; dull pain or discomfort in the middle or lower quadrants of the abdomen; general weakness and cold

2. Exhaustion of Intestinal Fluid

Exhaustion of Intestinal Fluid usually result from exhaustion of fluid and Blood in the whole body. It occurs in elderly people with deficiency of fluids, in post-partum with excessive blood loss, and in prolonged exogenous Heat disorders.

Syndrome: Symptoms:

Exhaustion of   persistent constipation; dry stools;
Intestinal Fluid   difficult bowel movements; mild abdominal
                               pain and distention or the absence of
                               prominent abdominal fullness or pain

   3.   Damp-Heat in the Large Intestine

This syndrome results from eating too much cold or raw food or eating contaminated food. The invasion of an exogenous pathogenic Heat can lead to the accumulation of Damp-Heat in the large intestine which obstructs the Qi and affects the function of transportation and absorption.

Syndrome: Symptoms:

Damp-Heat in the   diarrhea; abdominal pain;
Large Intestine   dark and foul-smelling stools; blood-tinged
                               mucus in the stool; burning sensation in the
                               anus

H.   The Urinary Bladder

The syndromes of the Urinary Bladder involve Damp-Heat in the Urinary Bladder and physiological dysfunction of the urinary bladder due to Deficient Kidney Yang.

Syndromes: Symptoms:

Damp-Heat in the   frequent urination; painful urination;
Urinary Bladder   hematourea

dysfunction of the   dribbling urination; weak stream of
Urinary Bladder due   urine; weakness of the lumbar area
to Deficient Kidney   and knees; intolerance to cold; pale
Yang   tongue with white coating

I. The Gall Bladder

The gall bladder functions in the digestive process by storing bile and excreting it into the intestines. The gall bladder and the liver are closely related both in physiological function and pathological dysfunction. Damp-Heat in the Gall Bladder, for example, is due to depression of the Qi of the Liver, Stagnation of the Qi of the Liver and Stasis of Liver Blood.

Syndrome: Symptoms:

Damp-Heat in the   bitter taste in the mouth; vomiting of
Gall Bladder   sour and bitter fluid; bright yellowish skin;
                       pain in the hypochondriac region; pain in the
                       right quadrant of the upper abdomen;
                       yellow and sticky tongue coating

Chapter VII

Differential diagnosis According to the

Six Exogenous Factors and Phlegm

CHAPTER VII. DIFFERENTIAL DIAGNOSIS ACCORDING TO THE SIX EXOGENOUS FACTORS AND PHLEGM

SYNDROMES OF WIND

There are two categories of Wind syndromes: exogenous Wind and endogenous Wind. Exogenous Wind occurs when the surface of the body is exposed to a pathogenic Wind which results in symptoms such as headache, nasal obstruction, sore throat and sweating. Endogenous Wind arises from internal pathogenic factors such as Liver Yang Ascending and transforming to Wind. The symptoms may include dizziness, tremors and convulsions. In the condition of Liver Wind stirred up by Heat, the symptoms of spasms, tremors of the four limbs and high fever would be present. If Deficient Liver Blood leads to Liver Wind, there will be itching of the skin.

A. Exogenous Pathogenic Wind

1. Wind-cold

This is an Exterior Cold syndrome. The patient has pronounced symptoms of headache, generalized body aches and pain, intolerance to cold, little or no sweating, cough with sputum that is clear and scanty, absence of thirst, the tongue is moist with a white coating, and the pulse is superficial and tight.

2. Wind-heat

This is an Exterior Heat syndrome. The symptoms of Wind-Heat include fever with or without the presence of sweating, intolerance to wind, headache, a pronounced cough with sputum that is sticky and yellow, redness and swelling of the tonsils, thirst, a red tongue, and a superficial and rapid pulse.

B. Pathogenic Wind Invades the Jing Luo (the channels and meridians)

There are three types of pathological manifestations:

1. Spasm of the local muscles and tendons and facial paralysis (Bell's Palsy).

2. Stiffness of the mouth, difficulty in opening the mouth, convulsions, rigidity of the trunk.

3. Bi-syndrome caused by pathogenic Wind, Cold and Damp. The clinical signs are pain or rigidity in the joints (either locally or through the whole body), and abnormal physical movement.

Concepts Basic to Syndromes of the Wind

A. Recognize the characteristics of pathogenic Wind.

1. With endogenous pathogenic Wind the patient not only has an exterior syndrome but also a syndrome of the upper respiratory tract.

2. Bi-syndrome due to pathogenic wind is characterized by pain that moves from one location to another and is not fixed in one specific area.

B. Pathogenic Wind often combines with another pathogenic factor.

1. Exogenous pathogenic wind is differentiated into Wind-Cold and Wind-Heat.

2. Skin disorders can be caused by Wind-Cold or Wind-Heat.

3. Bi-syndrome results from Wind, Cold and Damp.

C. Recognize the clinical significance of exogenous and endogenous Wind.

1. The disorders resulting from exogenous Wind are generally acute disorders.

2. The disorders resulting from endogenous Wind are usually chronic in nature. Endogenous Wind can occur in the course of a chronic or febrile disease .

D. The pulse in a Wind syndrome is usually superficial and rapid.

SYNDROMES OF COLD

Cold syndromes are differentiated into exogenous Cold and endogenous Cold. The exogenous Cold is caused by pathogenic Cold factor, from eating cold food or liquids, and from exposure to Cold weather. The syndrome of endogenous Cold occurs when the Yang Qi of the body is depleted and the body temperature is below normal. Endogenous and exogenous Cold are interrelated in that a Yang Deficiency can cause the patient to be vulnerable to attack by exogenous cold.

A. Exogenous pathogenic Cold

This condition usually occurs together with pathogenic Wind. The clinical manifestation of exogenous Cold are headache, intolerance to cold, cough or the absence of cough, clear and scanty sputum, the absence of thirst, pain in the joints, a white and moist tongue coating and a superficial, tight pulse.

B. Cold-Bi

Cold-Bi is a Bi-syndrome with more prominent cold symptoms. Bi-syndrome is caused by pathogenic Wind, Cold and Damp. The patient has symptoms of severe pain in the muscle and joints, abnormal physical movement or rigidity of the trunk or limbs.

C. Cold-Pain

This condition occurs from the over consumption of raw or cold food and attack by pathogenic Cold. The pain is sharp and it is associated with tension in the epigastrium. The pain is relieved by warmth and, conversely, becomes more severe with cold. The patient also has symptoms of vomiting with clear fluid, watery stools, coldness in the four limbs, a pale tongue proper with a white and moist coating, and a wiry and tight or deep and slow pulse.

Concepts Basic to Syndromes of Cold

A. Recognize the characteristics of the pathogenic Cold.

1. The "cold phenomenon" is the major clinical manifestation.

   2. The tongue proper is pale or slightly red with a white and
       moist coating.

   3. The pulse is usually wiry and tight or slow.

B. Recognize the associations with other pathogenic factors.

   1. Exogenous pathogenic Cold is often associated with
       pathogenic Wind.

   2. Pathogenic Cold is often associated with pathogenic
       Damp. It is based on a Damp-Cold syndrome with more
       prominent signs of a "Cold phenomenon".

C. Recognize that pathogenic Cold can transfer to Heat.

   1. In the case of a common cold due to Wind Cold, the Cold
       syndrome may have been eliminated but a Heat syndrome
       remains in the body. The patient has a fever and the tongue
       coating changes from pale and moist to yellow and dry.
       The absence of thirst becomes a symptom of increased
       thirst. This indicates that the pathogenic Cold has trans-
       formed into Heat.

   2. Bi-syndrome due to pathogenic Wind, Cold or Damp can
       transform into Heat-Bi with a clinical manifestation of
       severe pain and swelling of the joints.

D. Recognize the differentiation of exogenous and endogenous Cold.

   1. Exogenous Cold results from Wind-Cold. Damp-Cold or
       the over consumption of cold food. The major clinical
       manifestations are hyperactivity of pathogenic Cold,
       stiffness of the muscle and joints, a white and moist tongue
       coating, and a superficial and rapid pulse.

   2. Endogenous Cold arises from the weakness of the Yang Qi.
       The patient has Deficient syndrome with a white and
       slippery tongue coating and a deep and wiry pulse.

SYNDROMES OF EXCESSIVE HEAT, DEFICIENT HEAT, SUMMER DAMP AND SUMMER HEAT

A. Excessive Heat

The syndrome of Excessive Heat has a prominent "heat phenomenon". Its nature is that of Fire. Symptoms include a flushed face, restlessness, convulsions, fevers, intolerance to heat, heat sensations in the abdominal and thoracic areas, thirst with the desire to drink cold fluids, constipation and dry stools, a red tongue proper with a yellow coating and a wide, rapid pulse.

B. Deficient Heat

This is associated with Endogenous Heat due to Deficient Yin. The major clinical manifestations are insufficiency of Yin fluids, dry mouth and pharynx, flushed face, restlessness, insomnia, heat in the palms of the hands, soreness of the feet, interior heat sensations in the whole body, a cracked red tongue proper with little tongue coating, and a thin, rapid and feeble pulse.

C. Summer Damp

Pathogenic Heat and Dampness can occur together in a warm and rainy season. The clinical manifestations include prolonged lowered body temperature, general lassitude, poor appetite, chest fullness, nausea and vomiting, watery stools, clear, scanty urine, a sticky tongue coating, and a thin and superficial pulse.

D. Summer Heat

Pathogenic Summer Heat occurs only in the summer. It is due to exposure to blazing sun on hot days or staying in a hot room with poor ventilation. It is usually called "Summer Stroke" and the syndrome has a prominent "heat phenomenon".The clinical signs include a high fever, thirst, scanty urine, restlessness, convulsions, either the absence of sweat or copious sweating, fatigue, a dry tongue coating, and a wide, rapid pulse.

Concepts Basic to Syndromes of Excessive Heat, Deficient Heat, Summer Damp and Summer Heat

A. Recognize the differentiation between Excessive Heat (Fire), Stagnate Fire, Deficient Fire, and Flare-up of Fire.

1. Pathogenic Heat (Fire) usually has a syndrome of "heat phenomenon".

2. The syndrome with "heat phenomenon" is not always due to pathogenic Heat (Fire).

3. Stagnate Fire occurs when pathogenic Cold invades the body during the course of an exogenous Heat syndrome. Pathogenic Heat remains in the body and is the cause of symptoms such as sore throat, swelling in the pharynx area and rash. If the syndrome of pathogenic Cold transforms into Phlegm-Damp while the exogenous Heat syndrome is present, the clinical signs will be restlessness and chest fullness.

4. The syndrome of Deficient Heat (Fire) is not caused by exogenous pathogenic Heat (Fire) but by Deficient Yin. The treatment principle must include nourishing the Yin as well as clearing Heat.

5. Flare-up Fire is a fire due to deficient Yang. It usually occurs in the condition of the Collapse of the Yang due to extreme endogenous Cold. The patient has a syndrome of flushed face, restlessness, and desire to drink small amounts of water, panting and feeble breathing. The treatment in this case involves the tonification of the Yang rather than clearing the Heat. The Heat in this case is not true Heat nor is the deficiency a Yin Deficiency. It is a syndrome of the Collapse of the Yang.

B. Identify the characteristics of Heat (Fire) Syndromes in the internal organs:

1. Heart Fire presents with symptoms of restlessness and insomnia.

2. Liver Fire presents with symptoms of headache, anxiety, redness of the eyes, and the patient easily becomes angry.

3. Lung Fire presents with sputum that contains blood, coughing with blood, dry pharynx and nose bleeding.

4. Kidney Fire presents with high fever, dream-disturbed sleep, and urine that contains blood.

5. Stomach Fire presents with a foul smell in the mouth, toothache, and constipation.

SYNDROMES OF DAMP

Diseases caused by pathogenic Damp usually occur in the summer and autumn seasons when the climate is marked by humidity. Pathogenic Damp is differentiated into two categories: exogenous Damp and endogenous Damp. The former indicates that the patient has been exposed to a damp enviornment or climate; the later is caused by the dysfunction of the transformation of fluids by the Spleen due to Deficiency. The syndromes of exogenous and endogenous Damp have a mutual effect on each other. Exogenous Damp can cause injury to the Spleen resulting in an endogenous Damp condition, and the dysfunction of transformation of fluids of the Spleen can weaken the body's resistence to exogenous Damp.

Pathogenic Damp is associated with Wind, Cold and Heat, and combines to form the complex pathogenic factors of Bi-Syndrome, Damp-Cold, and Damp-Heat.

A. Interior Retention of Damp

In the condition of Interior Retention of Damp, the transformation and transportation functions of the Spleen and Stomach are impaired by the retention of Damp. This usually occurs in the summer season. The clinical signs are chest fulness, poor appetite, general lassitude, loose stool, scanty urine, mild fever, a sticky tongue coating, and a thin and superficial pulse. If a patient who presents with these symptoms also has a prominent "heat phenomenon" syndrome, it is attributed to Damp-Heat.

B. Damp-Heat

Damp-Heat can cause many diseases. The clinical manifestation not only reveals a "Damp phenomenon" but also has a "Heat phenomenon". The clinical signs include fever, chest fullness, abdominal distention, nausea and vomiting, poor appetite, thirst without the desire to drink, constipation or diarrhea, scanty, yellow urine, a sticky and yellow tongue coating, and a slippery and rapid pulse.

Concepts Basic to Damp Syndromes

A. Identify the location of the Damp Pathogenic Factor.

  1. Damp retained in the Upper Jiao: the clinical signs are heaviness of the head, chest fullness, epigastric fullness and distension and poor appetite.

  2. Damp retained in the Middle Jiao: the clinical signs are chest fullness, abdominal distension, indigestion, thirst without the desire to drink, watery stool, general lassitude, and a thick and sticky tongue coating.

  3. Damp moving downward to the Lower Jiao: the clinical sign is dark yellow urine with little volume.

B. Identify the differences between Cold-Damp and Damp-Heat.

  1. Cold-Damp is due to the inactivity of Spleen Yang in its function of transforming fluids. The symptoms are abdominal distension, diarrhea, edema, and copious sputum.

  2 Damp-Heat occurs as a consequence of the attack by Exogenous Pathogenic Damp, or from hyperactivity of Stomach Fire due to the overconsumption of oily or sweet food. The clinical signs are general lassitude, chest fullness, abdominal distension, and a sticky tongue coating.

Considering that Damp belongs to pathogenic Yin and Heat belongs to pathogenic Yang, it is important to determine whether the syndrome involves more pronounced Heat and less Damp or more Damp and less Heat.

SYNDROMES OF DRYNESS

The symptom of dryness is the clinical manifestation of the impairment of fluid and blood or attack by exogenous pathogenic dryness. The former belongs to endogenous dryness and the latter belongs to exogenous dryness. Endogenous dryness is more common and more severe than exogenous dryness.

A. Exogenous Dryness

Exogenous dryness occurs in a dry climate or the autumn season. The clinical signs are dry cough with little sputum or sticky sputum that is difficult expel, dryness of the throat, pharynx, larynx, lips, tongue and nose, nose bleeding, dry and cracked skin, and constipation.

B. Endogenous Dryness

Endogenous dryness can occur in any stage of exogenous Heat diseases with symptoms of high fever, excessive sweating, vomiting or excessive diarrhea. The clinical signs are thirst associated with excessive fluid intake, and a red and dry tongue proper. In the latter stages of exogenous Heat Syndromes, when the Yin is injured by Heat, the main clinical signs will be a damp, red tongue proper with no coating, thirst without the desire to drink water, dry mouth and pharynx, and convulsions. This syndrome is associated with Deficient Yin and it usually occurs in conditions of prolonged disease, excessive hemorrhages, and prolonged use of diuretic medication.

Concepts Basic to Syndromes of Dryness

A. Differentiate the syndromes of dryness according to location in the Upper, Middle and Lower Jiao (Tripple Warmer)

   1. The syndrome of pathogenic dryness that is retained in the Uper Jiao exhibits the main clinical sign of cough and is associated with the lung.

   2. Pathogenic dryness retained in the Middle Jiao has thirst as its main clinical sign and is associated with the stomach.

3. Pathogenic dryness retained in the Lower Jiao has dry
    stool or constipation as its main clinical sign . This
    syndrome is associated with the intestines, the liver or the
    kidney. Deficient Blood of the Liver and Kidney can result
    in the retention of pathogenic dryness in the Lower Jiao.

SYNDROMES OF PHLEGM

When the transformation, transportation and excretory functions of
the Lung, Spleen, Stomach and Kidney are impaired or when Heat
(Fire) injures the fluid of the body, the result is the production of
Phlegm or sputum. The fluid in the lung will transform to phlegm
when the Lung is attacked by exogenous pathogenic factors that dis-
turb its dispersing and descending function. Phlegm forms when the
Spleen and Stomach loose the function of transportation and transformation; phlegm also forms as a result of irregular food intake.
Deficient Kidney Yang will result in fluid moving upward and forming phlegm. Excessive mental strain leads to stagnant Qi transforming into fire, or interior Heat due to Deficient Yin forms phlegm.

The different types of syndromes of Phlegm are Damp Phlegm, Cold
Phlegm, Heat Phlegm, Dry Phlegm and Wind Phlegm.

A. Damp Phlegm

Damp Phlegm occurs in the condition of chronic respiratory inflammatory disease, for example, chronic bronchitis. The clinical signs
are cough with copious sputum, chest fullness, nausea and vomiting,
general lassitude, a sticky tongue coating, and a slippery pulse.

B. Cold Phlegm

Cold Phlegm occurs in conditions of chronic respiratory inflamatory
disease, for example, chronic bronchitis and asthma. The clinical signs
are coughing with white and clear sputum, cold in the four limbs,
syndromes of "cold phenomenon", a white and moist tongue coatiang
and a wiry pulse.

C. Heat Phlegm

Heat Phlegm occurs in conditions of various acute respiratory inflammatory disease or the acute, episodic attack stage of chronic respiratory inflammatory disease. The clinical signs are cough with yellow, sticky sputum, panting, fever, thirst, chest pain, a red tongue proper with a yellow coating, and a slippery and rapid pulse.

D. Wind Phlegm

Wind Phlegm often occurs in epilepsy. The patient not only has a Wind Syndrome but also has a syndrome of sputum with clinical signs such as suddenly falling down, coma, convulsions and foamy sputum.

E. Dry Phlegm

Dry Phlegm occurs in chronic respiratory inflammatory disease. The clinical signs are cough with sticky and scanty phlegm or sticky sputum with little blood, and dryness of the pharynx, lips and tongue.

Basic Concepts of Phlegm Syndromes

Phlegm is the product of a pathological factor, but after having been formed, it will itself become a pathogenic factor and affect the physiological functioning of the internal organs.

A. Color and Volume of the Phlegm

If the color is the phlegm is white and the volume copious, the syndrome is one of Dampness. If the phlegm is white and clear as well as copious, then the syndrome is one of Cold. A Heat syndrome presents with phlegm that is yellow and sticky and may be tinged with blood. If the phlegm is foamy, it indicates a Wind syndrome.

B. Common Clinical Characteristics of Phlegm Syndromes

    1. a sticky and slippery tongue coating

    2. a wiry and rolling (slippery) pulse

C. Recognize the relationship between the clinical manifestations of the Phlegm and the location of the Phlegm.

1. When Phlegm is retained in the lung the main symptom will be coughing and panting.

2. When Phlegm is retained in the heart the main symptoms will be palpitations and an agitated mind.

3. When Phlegm is retained in the stomach the main symptoms are nausea and vomiting.

4. When Phlegm is retained in the chest the main symptoms will be chest fullness, cough, panting, and pain in the hypochondriac region.

5. When Phlegm is retained in the Jing Luo (channels and collaterals) the result is scrofula.

6. When Phlegm is retained in the four limbs the main symptom is spasm in the four limbs.

Chapter VIII

Differential Diagnosis According to the Theory of Channels and Collaterals

(Taiyang, Yangming, Shaoyang, Taiyin, Shaoyin and Jueyin)

CHAPTER VIII. DIFFERENTIAL DIAGNOSIS ACCORDING TO THE THEORY OF CHANNELS AND COLLATERALS (Taiyang, Yangming, Shaoyang, Taiyin, Shaoyin and Jueyin)

The principles of differential diagnosis according to the theory of the channels and collaterals is described in the *Nei Jing (Esoteric Book or Inner Canon),* the first written record of Chinese medicine dating from 1,200-4,000 B.C. In the *Nei Jing,* the etiology, clinical manifestations, and pathology of exogenous Heat syndromes (both acute and chronic communicable diseases which result from bacteria or virus in modern medicine) are classified within six stages of disease: Yangming, Taiyang, Shaoyang, Taiyin, Shaoyin and Jueyin diseases (6-Channel syndrome). The former three are called the Three-Yang syndrome and the later three are called the Three-Yin syndrome.

Concepts Basic to Syndromes of the Taiyang, Yangming, Shaoyang, Taiyin, Shaoyin and Jueyin Syndromes (Six-Channel Syndrome).

A. **The clinical characteristics of the syndromes of the Six-Channel Syndrome**

1. Taiyang Syndrome: Exterior Cold
2. Yangming Syndrome: both Interior Heat and Excess
3. Shaoyang Syndrome: pathogenic factors that are semi-exterior and semi-interior in nature
4. Taiyin Syndrome: Cold injures Spleen Yang
5. Shaoyin Syndrome: weakness and deficiency of Heart and Kidney and general lassitude
6. Jueyin Syndrome: Interior deficiency and the complex combination of Cold and Heat

B. **Six-Channel Syndrome can be transferred and connected to each other.**

In general, the major clinical manifestations in the early and middle stages of exogenous Heat syndromes are Heat and Excessive syndromes due to sufficient levles of antipathogenic Qi. If the patient's antipathogenic Qi tends to decline and become weak during the process of the exogenous Heat syndrome, the clinical manifestation will show a syndrome of Cold and Deficiency, Deficient Heat, or a complex combination of both Cold and Heat. In the process of exogenous Heat, the Three-Yang Syndrome (Taiyang, Yangming and Shaoyang) usually occurs in the early stages of disease and the Three-Yin Syndrome (Taiyin, Shaoyin and Jueyin) in the latter stages.

1. Transferral of Channels

    Whereas the TaiYang Syndrome usually occurs at the onset of an exogenous Heat syndrome, it can quickly transfer to another channel. The following diagram describes the order of transferral of the Three-Yang syndrome:

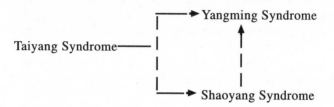

2. Combined Syndromes

    The order in which the Three-Yang Syndrome transfers to the other channels is not absolute because each patient maintains a different balance of antipathogenic and pathogenic Qi in the body. In general, when both the Shaoyang and the Yangming syndromes appear at the same time, it is called a "combined syndrome". The Shaoyang symptoms of intermittent Cold and Heat sensations, and pain and fullness in the chest and hypochondriac region combine with the Yangming symptoms of abdominal distension and pain, constipation, and a yellow tongue coating.

3. Two Sensation Syndrome

    In the Two Sensation syndrome, both Yin and Yang channel syndromes appear simultaneously. For example, the Taiyang syndrome and the Shaoyin syndrome appear together. The onset of the syndrome is marked by the clinical signs of fever and a deep pulse.

4. Occurring from the Original Channel

    The Taiyang syndrome usually transforms into the Yangming and Shaoyang syndromes. However, it may be that the disease process began with Yangming or Shaoyang symptoms and this is known as occurring from the original channel.

5. Directed Target

    The Three-Yin syndrome usually develops from the Three-Yang syndrome. In some cases, the Yin syndrome appears at the onset of disease and is known as the directed target.

    Therefore, the Six-Channel Syndrome can be viewed as a syndrome that has six different steps or as a syndrome that has six different prototypes. If the clinical picture changes from that of an exterior syndrome to an interior syndrome, or from Yang to Yin in nature, these indicate that the disease is progressing. If the clinical changes are from interior to exterior, or from Yin to Yang, these indicate that the disease is subsiding and the prognosis is positive.

TAIYANG SYNDROME

The Taiyang syndrome occurs when the body is invaded by an exogenous Heat factor. The major clinical signs are chills, intolerance to wind, headache, fever, soreness or pain in the body, neck stiffness, a thin, white and moist tongue coating and a superficial pulse.

A. Exterior Excess

This usually develops after an attack by exogenous Heat in a patient with a strong physical constitution. The clinical signs are absence of sweating, chills, and a superficial and rapid pulse.

B. Exterior Deficiency

This is usually seen in a patient with a weak physical constitution who is attacked by an exogenous Heat factor. The clinical signs are sweating, intollerance to wind and a superficial and slow pulse.

YANGMING SYNDROME

The Yangming Syndrome is marked by interior Heat and interior Excess syndromes. It is the clinical manifestation of the excessive Heat stage of the exogenous Heat syndrome. The clinical signs are fever, sweating, intolerance to heat, restlessness, thirst, abdominal distension and pain, constipation, a dry yellow tongue coating and a wide and rapid or deep and forceful pulse.

A. Yangming Channel Syndrome

The main clinical signs are high fever, excessive sweating, excessive thirst, and a wide and rapid pulse.

B. Yangming Organ Syndrome

The main clinical signs are fever, abdominal distension and discomfort with palpatory pressure, constipation, a dry yellow tongue coating, and a deep and forceful pulse.

SHAOYANG SYNDROME

The Shaoyang Syndrome occurs in patients with the condition of a weak antipathogenic factor on the exterior that permits movement of a pathogen to the interior where it stays in the Gall Bladder. The main clinical signs are intermittent sensations of cold and heat, pain and fullness in the hypochondriac region, decreased appetite, restlessness, nausea, a bitter taste in the mouth, dryness of the pharynx, dimmed vision, and a wiry pulse.

A. Shaoyang Syndrome conceals Exterior Syndrome

The main clinical signs are fever, intolerance to cold, and stiffness and pain in the joints.

B. Shaoyang Syndrome conceal Interior Syndrome

The main clinical signs are abdominal distension and pain and constipation.

C. Shaoyang syndrome conceal the Three-Yin Syndrome

This is a Deficiency syndrome.

TAIYIN SYNDROME

The Taiyin Syndrome is caused by the dysfunction of the transportation and transformation functions of the Spleen due to deficiency of Spleen Yang or weakness of Spleen Qi due to an attack by pathogenic Cold directly to the Taiyin channels.

Taiyin Syndrome and Yangming Organ Syndrome belong to the family of digestive tract disorders. The former syndrome is one of deficiency and the latter syndrome is one of excess. The clinical signs of the Taiyin Syndrome are abdominal pain, vomiting, diarrhea, indigestion, the absence of thirst, and a weak and slow pulse. The clinical signs of the Yangming Organ Syndrome are constipation, thirst, abdominal distension, and a deep and forceful pulse.

SHAOYIN SYNDROME

The Shaoyin Syndrome is caused by weakness and deficiency of the Kidney and Heart due to a weak physical constitution. The patient may have one of two different kinds of clinical symptomologies:

A. Deficient Cold

This is the most common condition of the Shaoyin Syndrome. The clinical signs are chills, general lassitute, sleepiness, coldness in the four limbs, mild diarrhea, and a feeble pulse.

B. Deficient Heat

This is caused by Deficient Kidney Yin and it is not often seen in the Shaoyin syndrome. The clinical signs are restlessness, insomnia, a dry mouth and pharynx, a dark red tongue proper, and a thin and rapid pulse.

JUEYIN SYNDROME

The Jueyin Syndrome results from an interior deficiency accompanied by a complex combination of Cold and Heat. The main clinical signs are heat in the upper part of the body and cold in the lower part of the body, thirst without the desire to drink water, hunger but no interest in eating, pain and sensations of heat in the area of the heart, cold in the four limbs, and various changes in the pulse.

PART TWO

METHODOLOGY OF

POINT PRESCRIPTIONS

It is essential that an acupuncturist be well-versed in traditional Chinese medical theory to perform an accurate diagnosis and point prescription. Without a precise diagnosis, a large number of points would be required in a point prescription in order to address each of the clinical symptoms.

The purpose of Part Two of this manual is to enhance your knowledge of Chinese medicine to effectively select points for prescriptions for various kinds of disorders. Just a few points, such as four to eight points, may be not only sufficient, but more effective than a prescription of ten or more points.

The following are the most important principles for prescribing and combining points in clinical practice.

A. Use of Essential Points

Each disease is associated with specific points that are the most effective in treatment. Acupuncture points have specific actions. For example, St 36 is the best point for treating stomach ulceration; GB 39 is chosen to treat neck stiffness; L.I. 4, Lu 7, St 36 and St 41 are all good for toothache, but L.I. 4 is the most effective. Therefore, it is important to understand the specific actions of each point in order to produce successful and remarkable results in each case.

B. An "Express Way"

The acupuncture point, or the area of responsiveness, is likened to a surface terminal station for the passage of disease. The points chosen have to be closely related to the location of the disease to facilitate the transfer of Qi directly and without interference. For example: GV 20, GB 20 and Yintang are located on the head and are selected in the treatment of mental disorders; Pc 6 , which acts directly on the chest, and CV 17, located on the sternum, are indicated in the treatment of chest pain or fullness and nausea or vomiting; Ht 7, Pc 6 and Ki 3 are for treating insomnia due to disharmony of the Heart and Kidney.

C. Fewer Points Create Less Interference

The use of not more than two points from the same meridian is a basic guideline for the point prescription. Some points on the same meridian will share the same indications and also may have the same needle sensation. The points in a prescription should address all of the clinical symptoms; however, too many points in a prescription may reduce the effectiveness of the treatment.

Secondly, certain points are useful in treating a broad range of symptoms. Those points that address a combination of symptoms in the clinical presentation are best in the point prescription. As an example, Sp 4 is not only chosen to treat frontal headache, but also to treat epigastric pain due to weakness of Spleen Yang.
UB 65 is effective in the treatment of occipital headache as well as back pain; UB 54 for constipation and back pain; Sp 10 for irregular menstruation and allergic itching.

Thirdly, the actions of some points may interfere with the actions of others in the same prescription. Some points can reduce the effectiveness of other points when used in combination. The point Pc 6, for example, is effective in regulating a rapid heart beat; but, based on clinical experience, it is less effective in reducing rapid heart beat with the addition of Ki 8 to the same prescription. Also, L.I. 4 is used to increase the movement and elasticity of the esophagus to relieve nausea, but when St 36 is added to the point prescription, this same action of L.I. 4 is diminished.

Chapter I

Concepts Basic to the Indications and

Prescriptions of the Essential Points

Among the Fourteen Meridians

CHAPTER I. CONCEPTS BASIC TO THE SPECIFIC
              INDICATIONS AND PRESCRIPTIONS OF THE
              ESSENTIAL POINTS AMONG THE FOURTEEN
              MERIDIANS

The physiological functions of each meridian are different from each other as are their indications. The following is an outline of the functions of each meridian according to the characteristics of each point on the meridian.

A. **The Lung Meridian (Lu)**

1. Activates the dispersing and descending functions of the Lung, resolves Phlegm, relieves cough and clears the lung.

    Main points are: Lu 11, Lu 10, Lu 9, Lu 5.

2. Removes obstruction from the channels and collaterals.

    Headache: Lu 7

3. Clear heat and relieve pain.

4. Stop bleeding

    a. hemoptysis: Lu 6, Lu 10, Lu 5
    b. nose bleeding: Lu 11

5. Pharyngitis: Lu 11, Lu 10, Lu 6

6. Epilepsy: Lu 11

B. **The Large Intestine Meridian (L.I.)**

1. Adjusts and regulates the gastro-intestinal system

    a. diarrhea: L.I. 11, L.I. 4
    b. abdominal pain: L.I. 4, L.I. 11

2. Disperses pathogenic heat of the Yangming channels:

  a. hypertension: L.I.11, L.I. 15
  b. epistaxis: L.I. 4, L.I. 1
  c. pharyngitis: L.I. 4, L.I. 1
  d. fever without sweating: L.I. 1, L.I. 4, L.I. 11

 3. Relieves pain

  Red eyes: L.I.1, L.I. 4

 4. Sedation

  Hysteria: L.I.4

 5. Relieves the exterior and clears the lung

  a. common cold: L.I.4, L.I. 11
  b. relieves cough and stops asthma: L.I.4, L.I. 1, L.I. 7

C. The Stomach Meridian (St)

 1. Adjusts and regulates the Spleen and Stomach

  a. stomachache: St 36, St 34
  b. abdominal pain: St 34, St 37
  c. diarrhea: St 25, St 43
  d. constipation: St 40, St 36, St 25
  e. vomiting: St 44, CV 12
  f. indigestion: St 36, St 25 (needle and moxa)

 2. Harmonizes Qi and Blood

  a. regulates Qi (cough, asthma): St 40, St 36
  b. regulates menstruation (irregular menstrual cycle; leukorrhea): St 25, St 44
  c. Decrease blood pressure: St 40, St 36
  d. Tachycardia: St 32

 3. Removes obstruction from the channels and collaterals, resolves Phlegm and eliminates Damp

  a. frozen shoulder: St 38

      b.   frontal headache: St 44
      c.   shoulder and back pain: St 31
      d.   sputum due to Phlegm-Damp: St 40

4.   Tonifies body constitution

      a.   headache due to deficiency of blood: St 44, St 36
      b.   weakness of body constitution: St 36

D. The Spleen Meridian (Sp)

1.   Regulates Spleen and Stomach

      a.   abdominal pain; diarrhea: Sp 4, Sp 6, Sp 9, Sp 3
      b.   constipation: Sp 3, Sp 5
      c.   vomiting: Sp 1, Sp 2
      d.   indigestion: Sp 4, Sp 6 (needle and moxa)

2.   Diuresis and eliminates Damp

      a.   edema: Sp 6, Sp 9
      b.   nocturnal enuresis: Sp 6, Sp 9, Sp 8

3.   Supports Spleen Yang and dominates blood

      a.   anemia: Sp 6, Sp 10 (needle and moxa)
      b.   menorrhagia : Sp 1, Sp 6, Sp 10
      c.   epistaxis, uremia, blood in the stool: Sp 1

4.   Removes obstruction from the channels and collaterals

      a.   weakness of the four limbs: Sp 21
      b.   numbness of the lower limbs: Sp 10
      c.   strong armpit odor: Sp 21

5.   Strengthens the Spleen, eliminates Damp and activates Blood

      a.   Headache due to phlegm damp: Sp 4, Sp 6, Sp 9
      b.   lumbar pain due to Cold-Damp: Sp 4, Sp 8, Sp 10

E. The Heart Meridian (Ht)

1. Sedates and Calms the mind

    Main points: Ht 7, Ht 3, Ht 6

2. Clears and disperses Heart Fire

    a. insomnia: Ht 6, Ht 8
    b. feverish sensations in the palms of the hand: Ht 6, Ht 8

3. Nourishes Heart Yin

    Night sweats: Ht 6

F. The Small Intestine Meridian (S.I.)

1. Disperses fire (sedative)

    a. epilepsy: S.I. 3, S.I. 7
    b. hysteria: S.I. 3, S.I. 7
    c. ringing in the ear (tinnitus): S.I. 3, S.I. 19
    d. night sweats: S.I. 3

2. Relieves pain

    a. shoulder pain: S.I. 3, S.I.9, S.I. 11
    b. toothache: S.I. 18, S.I. 19
    c. headache: S.I. 1, S.I. 3, S.I. 7
    d. pharyngitis: S.I.1

G. The Urinary Bladder Meridian (UB)

1. Disperses pathogenic heat

    a. eye disorders: UB 1, UB 18
    b. benefits the Liver and Gall Bladder
        1) hepatitis: UB 18, UB 19
        2) bitter taste in the mouth: UB 19
        3) choledochitis : UB 18, UB 19

    c.   detoxification: UB 54
    d.   hemorrhoids: UB 54, UB 57

2. Relieves exterior Heat

    a.   common cold: UB 12, UB 13
    b.   cough: UB 11, UB 12, UB 13
    c.   asthma: UB 11, UB 12, UB 13, UB 23

3. Regulates Spleen and Stomach

    a.   stomachache: UB 18, UB 19, UB 20, UB 21
    b.   vomiting: UB 17, UB 20, UB 21
    c.   hiccough: UB 17, UB 21
    d.   diarrhea: UB 20, UB 21, UB 23, UB 25
    e.   constipation: UB 22, UB 25, UB 28
    f.   abdominal distention: UB 20, UB 25, UB 22, UB 21

4. Nourishes Kidney Yin

    a.   night sweats: UB 13, UB 14, UB 43
    b.   tinnitus: UB 22, UB 23, UB 19

5. Diuresis and relieves edema

    a.   retention of urine: UB 23
    b.   edema: UB 20, UB 22, UB 23
    c.   nocturnal enuresis: UB 23, UB 28

6. Regulates menstruation; relieves pain

    a.   irregular menstruation: UB 60, UB 67, UB 23
    b.   lumbago: UB 23, UB 28, UB 54, UB 57, UB 60
    c.   occipital headache: UB 60, UB 65
    d.   paralysis in the lower limbs: UB 54, UB 57, UB 60

7. Sedative and calm mind.

    a.   hysteria: UB 15, UB 20
    b.   epilepsy: UB 15, UB 27, UB 18, UB 62, UB 63
    c.   impotence: UB 23, UB 26

    d. dizziness: UB 10, UB 62

    e. anxiety : UB 15, UB 14, UB 44

H. The Kidney Meridian (Ki)

    1. Nourishes Kidney Yin

        a. tinnitus: Ki 3, Ki 7

        b. toothache: Ki 3

        c. nephritis: Ki 3, Ki 7

        d. irregular menstruation: Ki 2, Ki 3, Ki 5, Ki 6

        e. night sweats: Ki 7

        f. hypertension: Ki 1

    2. Warms Kidney Yang

        a. retention of urine: Ki 1, Ki 5, Ki 6, Ki 10

        b. edema: Ki 7, Ki 3

        c. diarrhea: Ki 2, Ki 3, Ki 7

        d. lumbago: Ki 3, Ki 7

    3. Harmonizes Kidney and Heart (sedative)

        a. hysteria: Ki 1, Ki 4, Ki 6

        b. insomnia: Ki 3

        c. anxiety: Ki 3

I. The Pericardium Meridian (Pc)

    1. Harmonizes stomach function

        a. vomiting: Pc 6, Pc 3

        b. abdominal pain: Pc 7, Pc 6

        c. stomachache: Pc 6, Pc 7, Pc 3

    2. Nourishes Yin

    Night sweats: Pc 4, Pc 5

3. Disperses Heart Fire

    a. hysteria: Pc 4, Pc 6
    b. tachycardia: Pc 4, Pc 5, Pc 6
    c. anxiety: Pc 4, Pc 5, Pc 6, Pc 7
    d. foul mouth odor: Pc 7
    e. heat in the palms of the hand: Pc 8, Pc 9
    f. fever without sweating : Pc 3, Pc 5, Pc 6, Pc 9
    g. epistaxis: Pc 4

4. Regulates Qi in the Upper Jiao (chest area)

    a. asthma: Pc 6
    b. hiccough: Pc 6

J. The Triple Warmer Meridian (TW)

1. Regulates the Spleen and Stomach

    a. abdominal pain: TW 4, TW 5
    b. diarrhea: TW 6
    c. constipation: TW5, TW 6
    d. vomiting: TW 5
    e. reduces cholesterol levels: TW 6

2. Disperses Heat and relieves pain

    a. frontal headache: TW 1, TW 23
    b. intercostal neuralgia: TW 6
    c. migraine headache: TW 2, TW 3, TW 4, TW 23
    d. painful upper limbs: TW 2, TW 3, TW 5, TW 6
    e. painful lower limbs: TW 5, TW 6

3. Disperses the Fire of the Triple Warmer

    a. tinnitus: TW 2, TW 3, TW 5, TW 6, TW 17, TW 21
    b. deafness: TW 3, TW5
    c. anxiety : TW 1, TW 2
    d. fever without sweating: TW 1, TW 2, TW 3, TW 5, TW 6
    e. great thirst: TW4

K. The Gall Bladder Meridian (GB)

1. Disperses liver and gall bladder heat

    a. migraine headache: GB 20, GB 39, GB 34, GB 31
    b. intercostal neuralgia: GB 34, GB 15, GB 44
    c. toothache: GB 2
    d. sciatica: GB 31, GB 39
    e. sinus problems: GB 20, GB 34
    f. hepatitis: GB 34, GB 39
    g. mumps: GB 20
    h. hypertension: GB 20, GB 39
    i. epistaxis: GB 20, GB 39
    j. tinnitus: GB 20, GB 21, GB 43

2. Regulates menstruation and relieves leukorrhea

    a. irregular menstruation: GB 26
    b. leukorrhea: GB 20, GB 26

3. Activates Blood and relieves Blood Stasis

    a. lumbar pain due to Blood Stasis: GB 31, GB 21
    b. stomachache due to Blood Stasis: GB 34, GB 24, GB 40, GB 15
    c. intercostal neuralgia due to Blood Stasis: GB 34, GB 40

L. The Liver Meridian (Liv)

1. Disperses Liver fire and regulates Qi

    a. menorrhagia: Liv 1, Liv 3
    b. irregular menstruation: Liv 3, Liv 5
    c. parietal headache: Liv 2, Liv 3
    d. Intercostal neuralgia: Liv 3, Liv 13, Liv 14
    e. hernia: Liv 1, Liv 3, Liv 8
    f. epilepsy : Liv 1, Liv 3, Liv 8

2. Disperses Liver and Gall Bladder Heat

    a. hypertension : Liv 3
    b. hepatitis: Liv 2, Liv 3, Liv 4
    c. nephritis: Liv 8
    d. jaundice: Liv 3, Liv 4, Liv 13, Liv 14
    e. glaucoma: Liv 2, Liv 3
    f. anxiety; anger: Liv 3

M. The Conception Vessel Meridian (CV)

1. Regulates menstruation

    a. irregular menstruation: CV 3, CV 4, CV 6
    b. menorrhagia: CV 3, CV 4
    c. leukorrhea: CV 3, CV 6, CV 5
    d. menostasia: CV 4, CV 5, CV 6

2. Regulates the Spleen and Stomach

    a. indigestion: CV 12, CV 13
    b. diarrhea: CV 12, CV 5, CV 4, CV 9
    c. constipation: CV 12, CV 6, CV 4
    d. stomachache: CV 12, CV 13, CV 10
    e. hiccough: CV 4, CV 12, CV 17

3. Relieves cough and moves Qi of the Upper Jiao

    a. cough: CV 17, CV 22
    b. asthma: CV 17, CV 22

4. Strengthens body constitution

Main points: CV 4, CV 6, CV 12

N. The Governing Vessel Meridian (GV)

1. supports Yang Qi

    a. headache due to Deficient Yang Qi: GV 20, GV 16, GV 23, GV 24
    b. stroke: GV 20

2. clears Heat

    a. jaundice: GV 14, GV 13, GV 9
    b. fever: GV 14, GV 13

3. Sedates and calms the mind

    Main points: GV 22, GV 20, GV 26, GV 16

4. Polyurea or oligurea: GV 4

5. Harmonizes Qi and Blood

    a. epistaxis: GV 20, GV 16, GV 23
    b. hypertension: GV 20
    c. anemia: GV 14, GV 9
    d. irregular menstruation: GV 4, GV 3
    e. leukorrhea: GV 4
    f. oligoleukocytosis (leukopenia): GV 14

Chapter II

The Most Commonly Used Points

and Their Indications

CHAPTER II THE MOST COMMONLY USED POINTS AND THEIR INDICATIONS

There are 365 points on the 14 meridians; however, only about 46 points have been commonly used in Chinese acupuncture dating from ancient times through to today. Although only 46 points are generally used, these points are especially effective and produce remarkable results. These successful results are dependent on the Chinese diagnosis, the point prescription and the skilful application of acupuncture technique by the acupuncturist.

The 46 main points are divided into three classes. The 12 points in the first class are the most commonly used points. The second class is a group of 25 points that are used most commonly after the first class of points. The other 9 points belong to third class.

The symbols included in this chapter are:

SYMBOL   MEANING

_/_   the needle is inserted in the one side of the body (laterally)

_||_   the needles are inserted on both sides (bilaterally)

I/   blood letting instead of needle insertion

_^_   moxibusion

A. THE FIRST CLASS POINTS — the most commonly used points.

1. FENG SHI/GB31

Location: On the midline of the lateral aspect of the thigh, 7 cun above the transverse politeal crease.

Indications:

a.   One of the most important points for use in sedation.

b. Especially effective for painful disorders of the lateral
    side of the body such as: migraine headaches, shoulder
    and back pain, costal pain, rheumatism of the lower
    limbs, and sciatica. _/_

2. SHU GU/UB 65

Location: On the lateral side of the dorsum of the foot, posterior and
inferior to the head of the fifth metatarsal bone, at the junction of the
red and white skin.

Indications:

A. Especially effective in the treatment of:

    a   occipital headache _II_
    b. neck pain and stiffness _/_
    c. parietal headache _II_

B. Commonly used for the treatment of:

    a. back pain _/_
    b. low back and lumbar pain _/_

Note: This point is effective for painful disorders of the posterior
part of the body.

3. GONG SUN/ SP 4

Location: In the depression distal and inferior to the base of the first
metatarsal bone, at the junction of the red and white skin.

Indications:

This point is effective for various disorders of the interior part of the
body.

    a. frontal headache

    b. soreness and pain of the nasal bone and infra-orbital
        region

    c.   various disorders of the Spleen and Stomach (very effective for gastric ptosis)

    d.   hypertension _||_

    e.   numbness of the hand _||_

4.   WEI ZHONG/UB 54

Location: Midpoint of the transverse crease of the poplitial fossa between the tendons of m. biceps femoris and m. semitendinosus.

Indications:

    a.   physical injury in the lumbar region I/

    b.   pain in the heel I/

    c.   pain in the ankle

    d.   hemorrhoids I/

    e.   asthma (with Lu 5) I/

    f.   pain in the low back, scrofulosis and furuncle, venereal disease I/

    g.   severe occipital headache and neck pain I/

    h.   brain concussion

    i.   sciatica (with Hou Xi, S.I 3, Wan Gu, S.I 4 after blood letting of UB 54) I/

    j.   cholera (with Chi Ze, Lu 5) I/

    k.   varix of the women (insert the needle at Nei Guan, Pc 6, Tai Yuan, and Lu 9 after blood letting of UB 54)

5. HOU XI/ S.I. 3

Location: When a loose fist is made, the point is proximal to the head of the fifth metacarpal bone on the ulnar side, in the depression at the junction of the red and white skin.

Indications:

      a.   lumbar and lumbar vertebral pain _/_

      b.   neck stiffness _/_

      c.   sciatica (with Shu Gu, UB 65) _/_

      d.   shoulder pain _/_

      e.   backache

      f.   leg pain when bending or twitching of the leg _/_

6. NEI GUAN/ Pc 6

Location: 2 cun above the transverse crease of the wrist, between the tendons of m. palmaris longus and m. flexor carpi radialis.

Indications:

      a.   various disorders of the heart _||_

      b.   chest fullness and pain _||_

      c.   knee pain _||_

      d.   numbness of the middle finger _||_

      e.   neck stiffness _||_

      f.   pain on the interior side of the leg _||_

      g.   asthma _||_

    h.   stomach disorders (with Gong Sun, Sp 4) _||_

    i.   night sweating _||_

7. YEMEN/TW 2

Location: Proximal to the margin of the web between the ring and small fingers. The point is located with a clenched fist.

Indications:

    a.   fatigue _||_

    b.   tired eyes _/_

    c.   leg pain _/_

    d.   sore throat (with Yu Ji, Lu 10) _/_

    e.   chest fullness

8. LIANG QUI/St 34

Location: 2 cun above the laterosuperior border of the patella.

Indications:

    a.   stomach ache, stomach ulceration, gastrorrhagia and various gastro-intestinal disorders _||_

    b.   abdominal pain _||_

    c.   breast pain _/_

    d.   pain in the upper part of the chest _/_

9. TIAO KOU/ St 38

Location: 8 cun below Dubi (St 35), 2 cun below Shang Ju Xu (St 37) and Jie Xi (St 41).

Indications:

    a. shoulder and back pain

    b. elbow pain

    c. pain in index finger

10. CHI ZE/ Lu 5

Location: On the cubital crease, on the radial side of the tendon of m. biceps brachii.

Indications: Especially effective for:

  A. Seven Star Needle

    a. asthma (with Wei Zhong, UB 54)

    b. chest fullness and pain

    c. unable to raise the shoulders and arm; aching of the shoulder and arm

    d. cholera (with Wei Zhong, UB 54)

    e. pain in the wrist

  B. Needle insertion

    a. hemiplegia _/_

    b. frequent urination _||_

    c. motor impairment of any joint

11. QU CHI/ L.I. 11

Location: When the elbow is flexed, the point is in the depression at the lateral end of the transverse cubital crease.

Indications:

    a. dizziness

    b. hyper- or hypotension

    c. rhinitis; conjunctivitis; acne

    d. skin disorders

    e. acute dysentery

12. SAN YIN JIAO/ Sp 6

Location: 3 cun directly above the tip of the medial malleolus (the ankle), on the posterior border of the tibia.

Indications:

    a. obstetrical and gynecological disorders

    b. disorders of the kidney (with Yin Ling Quan, Sp 9)

    c. diabetes (with SP9)

    d. impotence

    e. fullness in the lower part of the abdomen (with St 36)

    f. insomnia (with Shemmen, Ht 7)

    g. lumbar vertebral pain; neck stiffness

B. THE SECOND CLASS POINTS

13. YING LING QUAN/Sp 9

Location: On the lower border of the medial condyle of the tibia in the depression between the posterior border of the tibia and m. gastrocnemius.

Indications:

    a.   frontal headache; headache; aching of the nasal bone

    b.   acute and chronic diarrhea (with Qu Chi, L.I. 11)

    c.   diabetes (with San Yin Jiao, Sp 6)

    d.   kidney disorders nephrotic edema (with Fu Liu, Ki 7)

    e.   hyperactivity of the gastric juices; nausea

    f.   retention of urine (with St 36)

14. ZU SAN LI/St 36

Location: 3 cun below Dubi (St 35) one finger-breadth from the anterior crest of the tibia.

Indications:

    a.   gastro-intestinal disorders including ulceration of the stomach; acute gastro-intestinal inflammation _II_; loss of appetite _II_; vomiting _II_; indigestion _II_; diarrhea _II_

    b.   hypertrophic rhinitis (with Ying Xiang, L.I. 20) _II_

    c.   toothache _II_

    d.   spasm

    e.   chronic disorders of the stomach, chest fullness (Seven Star Needle)

15. HE GU/ LI 4

Location: Between the 1st and 2nd metacarpal bones, approximately at the mid-point of the 2nd metacarpal bone on the radial side.

Indications:

    a.   toothache (with St 36)

    b.   rhinitis _/_

    c.   elbow pain

    d.   asthma (with Sp 6) _ll_

    e.   scrofulosis and furnuncle (with L.I. 11) _ll_

    f.   facial and eye disorders (with L.I 11)

    g.   acute tonsillitis (with Shao Shang, Lu 11)

16. BI GUAN/St 31

Location: Directly below the anterior superior iliac spine, in the depression on the lateral side of m. sartorius when the thigh is flexed.

Indications:

    A.   Especially effective for:

        a.   pain in the thigh

        b.   pain in the neck and back

    B.   Commonly effective in the treatment of:

        a.   obstetrical disorders

        b.   common cold

17. XIAN GU/St 43

Location: In the depression distal to the junction of the 2nd and 3rd metatarsal bones.

Indications:

    a.   migraine headache _/_

    b.   diarrhea

    c.   abdominal distension (with Nei Ting, St 44 _||_ , St 36 _||_, and Sp 6 _||_)

18. NEI TING/St 44

Location: Proximal to the web margin between the 2nd and 3rd toes, in the depression distal and lateral to the 2nd metatarsodigital joint.

Indications:

    a.   dysmenorrhea _||_

    b.   menorrhagia

    c.   rubella _||_

    d.   difficult labor (contraindicated for pregnant women) _||_

19. FU TU/St 32

Location: 6 cun above the laterosuperior border of the patella, on the line connecting the anterior superior iliac spine and the lateral border of the patella.

Indications:

    a.   cardiac and hematological disorders _||_

    b.   pain in the four limbs

    c.   edema in lower extremities

20. CHENG SHAN/UB 57

Location: Directly below the belly of m. gastrocnemius, on the line connecting Wei Zhong (UB 54) and the tendo-calcaneus, about 8 cun below UB 54.

Indications:

    A. Especially effective for:

        Lumbar and back pain _ll_

    B. Commonly effective for:

        a. anal fistula (with Lu 7 after blood-letting of UB 57)

        b. sports injury

        c. muscle spasms

21. KUN LUN/ UB 60

Location: In the depression between the external malleolus and tendo-calcaneus.

Indications:

        a. vertebral pain (especially effective) _ll_

        b. diarrhea before sunrise _ll_

        c. ankle swelling and pain _ll_

22. SHEN MAI/UB 62

Location: In the depression directly below the external malleolus.

Indications:

        a. heel pain _/_

        b. sciatica

23. FU LIU/Ki 7

<u>Location</u>: 2 cun directly above Tai Xi, Ki 3, on the anterior border of tendo-calcaneus.

<u>Indications</u>:

      a.   various disorders due to Kidney Deficiency

      b.   low back pain (with Hou Xi, S.I. 3) _||_

      c.   numbness of the hand _||_

      d.   eye disorders

      e.   edema and Cold and Damp disorders

24. ZHANG ZHU/TW 3

<u>Locations</u>: When the hand is placed with the palm facing downward, the point is on the dorsum of hand between the 4th and 5th metacarpal bones, in the depression proximal to the metacarpophalangeal joint.

<u>Indications</u>:

      a.   low back pain _/_

      b.   pain in the upper limbs

      c.   pain in the neck, back and shoulder

      d.   rheumatoid arthritis (with Yemen, TW 2)

25. ZHI GOU/TW 6

<u>Location</u>: 3 cun above Yang Chi, TW 4, between the ulna and radius.

<u>Indications</u>:

      a.   chest fullness _||_

b.   intercostal neuralgia _/_

c.   pain in the forearm

d.   constipation (especially effective) _ll_

26. YANG LING QUAN/ GB 34

Location: In the depression interior and inferior to the head of the fibula.

Indications:

a.   hypochondriac pain (very effective) _ll_

b.   hemorrhage of the internal organs _ll_

c.   motor impairment of various joints

d.   upper limb pain

e.   migraine headache

f.   trigeminal neuralgia

g.   wrist pain

27. XUAN ZHONG/ GB 39

Location: 3 cun above the tip of the external malleolus in the depression between the posterior border of the fibula and the tendons of m. peronaeus longus and brevis.

Indications:

a.   pain in coccygeal bone (very effective) _/_

b.   neck stiffness _/_

c.   various disorders of the bone marrow

d.   ankle injury _/_

28. XIA XI/GB 43

Location: Between the 4th and 5th toes, proximal to the margin of the web.

Indications:

    a.   dizziness; blurred vision (with Qu Chi, L.I 11)

    b.   febrile disorders

29. TAI CHONG/Liv 3

Location: In the depression distal to the junction of the 1st and 2nd metatarsal bones.

Indications:

Effective for various excessive syndromes of the liver meridian.

    a.   hypertension

    b.   hyperactivity of gastric juices

    c.   stomachache or disharmonious Stomach Qi

    d.   hemorrhagia nasali (epistaxis)

    e.   neurasthenia

    f.   nightmare

    g.   hand or foot pain (with He Gu, L.I. 4)

30. QU QUAN/Liv 8

Location: On the medial side of the knee joint.

Indications:

    a.   ptosis of the uterus (very effective)

    b.   cystitis; gonorrhea

31. GUAN YUAN/CV 4

Location: On the midline of the abdomen, 3 cun below the umbilicus.

Indications:

    a.   various disorders caused by Kidney Deficiency

    b.   impotence

    c.   premature ejaculation _^_

32. QI HAI/CV 6

Location: On the midline of the abdomen, 1.5 cun below the umbilicus.

Indications:

    a.   various disorders caused by Kidney Deficiency

    b.   irregular menstruation

33. ZHONG WAN/CV 12

Location: On the midline of the abdomen, 4 cun above the umbilicus.

Indications:

    a.   frontal headache

    b.   general tonification headache treatment

    c.   gastro-enteritis; gastric ptosis; stomachache

d.   diabetes (with Yin Ling Quan, Sp 8)

34. SHAN ZHONG/CV 17

<u>Location</u>: On the midline of the sternum, between the nipples, level with the 4th intercostal space.

<u>Indications</u>:

a.   asthma

b.   various Qi deficient disorders (with Pc 6)

c.   various Qi excessive disorders (with Liv 3)

35. DA ZHUI/GV 14

<u>Location</u>: Between the spinous processes of the 7th cervical vertebra and the 1st thoracic vertebra approximately at the level of the shoulder.

<u>Indications</u>:

a.   various febrile disorders (i.e. tonsillitis)

b.   parasitic diseases

c.   malaria

36. REN ZHONG/GV 26

<u>Location</u>: Below the nose, slightly above the midpoint of the philtrum.

<u>Indications</u>:

a.   for emergency cases, to revive consciousness

b.   pain in the lumbar vertebra (with UB 60)

c.   swelling of the face

37. BAI HUI/GV 20

Location: 7 cun above the posterior hairline, on the midpoint of the line connecting the apexes of the two auricles.

Indications:

    a.   CVA (cerebral vascular accident); hypertension

    b.   headache

    c.   ptosis of the organs _^_

    d.   hemiplegia

C. THE THIRD CLASS POINTS

38. KONG ZUI/Lu 6

Location: On the palmar aspect of the forearm, on the line joining Tai Yuan (Lu 9) and Chize (Lu 5).

Indications:

    Bleeding hemorrhoids (with Cheng Shan, UB 57, after blood letting of UB 54)

39. LIE QUE/Lu 7

Location: Superior to the styloid process of the radius, 1.5 cun above the transverse crease of the wrist.

Indications:

    a.   ache in the whole head (with Chi Yin, UB 67)

    b.   dysuria

    c.   pain in testes or vagina

    d.   blood stasis in chest resulting from physical injury (Seven Star Needle)

40. YU JI/Lu 10

Location: On the radial aspect of the midpoint of the 1st metacarpal bone, at the junction of the red and white skin (the junction of the dorsum and palm of the hand).

Indications:

     a.   stomach ache _/_

     b.   abnormal stool _/_

     c.   sore throat (with Yemen, TW 2): very effective _/_

     d.   pain in palm of hand

41. SHAO SHANG/Lu 11

Location: On the radial side of the thumb approximately 0.1 cun posterior to the corner of the nail.

Indications:

     a.   for emergency febrile cases (bloodletting)

     b.   sore throat or tonsillitis l/

     c.   hemorrhagia nasali (epistaxis)

     d.   febrile diseases l/

42. SHANG YANG/L.I 1

Location: On the radial side of the index finger approximately 0.1 cun posterior to the corner of the nail.

Indications:

     a.   sore throat

     b.   emergency febrile cases l/

c. febrile diseases

43. SHOU SAN LI/L.I 10

Location: 2 cun below Qu Chi, L.I. 11.

Indications:

a. shoulder and back pain _|_

b. ear pain (with Tai Xi, KI 3)

c. scrofulosis and furuncle

d. rhinitis (sinusitis) with L.I. 4, L.I. 20, L.I. 11

44. YING XIANG/L.I. 20

Location: In the nasolabial groove at the level of the midpoint of the lateral border of ala nasi.

Indications:

a. sinusitis

b. acne

c. facial itching

45. FENG LONG/St 40

Location: 8 cun superior and anterior to the external malleolus about one finger-breadth posterior to Tiao Gou (St 38).

Indications:

a. excessive sputum: very effective _||_

b. hypertension |/

c. acute gastro-enteritis _||_

46. SHENMEN/Ht 7

<u>Location</u>: On the transverse crease of the wrist, in the articular re-
gion between the pisiform bone and the ulna, in the depression on the
radial side of the tendon of m. flexor carpi ulnaris.

<u>Indications</u>:

      a.   insomnia: very effective when used with San Yin Jiao,
           Sp 6

      b.   epilepsy (with Feng Fu, GV 16)

      c.   sedation

      d.   neurasthenia (with San Yin Jiao, Sp 6)

Chapter III

Methods for Point Prescription

and Combination

CHAPTER III. METHODS FOR POINT PRESCRIPTION AND COMBINATION

There are many approaches to point selection in clinical practice. In this chapter each method for governing the prescription and combination of points will be discussed in terms of the differential diagnosis, the functions of the meridians, the characteristics and indications of the points, and the theory of Chinese medical science. Through the point selection process, a point prescription is derived that can result in a better and more remarkable result in treatment.

A. The Generally Applied Prescribing Method

Local points or adjacent points are selected to treat the affected region of the body.

1. Head: St 8; GV 20; GB 20

2. Chest: Pc 6; CV 17

3. Upper limbs: L.I. 11; L.I. 10; L.I. 4

4. Lower limbs: GB 34; GB 30

5. Hypochondriac and Costal regions: TW 6; GB 34; Liv 13

6. Upper Abdomen: CV 12; CV 13; St 36; St 43

7. Lower Abdomen: CV 21; CV 13; St 36; Pc 6

8. Back: S.I. 11; UB 11; GV 14

9. Lower back: UB 23; UB 54; GB 30

The following prescription formula enhances the therapeutic effect:

1. Acute and Excessive syndromes: In addition to local and adjacent points, the points located on the four limbs are indicated for use according to the associated syndromes.

2. Chronic, Deficient and Cold syndromes: In addition to

local and adjacent points, the Back-Shu points are indicated for use according to the syndromes; the application of moxibustion in particular is effective.

B. The Single Point Applied Prescribing Method:

It requires only one specific point to effectively treat a certain syndrome or disease.

1. Anemia with dizziness: apply moxa stick over GV 20

2. Convulsion in children: Yintang

3. Coma: GV 26

4. Nasal bleeding (rhinorrhea): Apply moxa stick over GV 23

5. Frontal headache: Sp 4

6. Occipital or Partial Headache: UB 65

7. Migraine headache: GB 31

8. Neck stiffness: GB 39

9. Stomachache: St 34

10. Fever: GV 14 or L.I. 11

C. The Double Points Side-by-Side Prescribing Method

By this method, points are chosen bilaterally for treating certain diseases to enhance the therapeutic effect.

1. Chest pain or fullness: PC 6 or St 40

2. Lumbago: UB 23 or UB 54

3. Stomachache: St 34, St 36, or Sp 4

4. Sore throat: Lu 11 or L.I. 4

5. Dysmenorrhea: Sp 10 or Sp 6

6. Headache with neck stiffness: Lu 7, S.I. 3 or S.I. 11

7. Abdominal pain: St 38

8. Irregular heart beat: St 32

9. Intercostal neuralgia: GB 34

10. Neck stiffness: GB 39

11. Phlegm syndromes: St 40

D. The Four Limbs Mutual Prescribing Method

Use of the points on the four limbs is required to adjust the physiological functions of the internal organs and, specifically, for treating certain syndromes and diseases.

1. Stomachache with nausea and vomiting: Pc 6 and Sp 4

2. Gall Bladder diseases and costal neuralgia: TW 6 and GB 34

3. Toothache, sore throat: L.I. 4 and St 44

4. Parietal headache, insomnia, hypertension: L.I. 4 and Liv 3 or UB 54 and Pc 3

5. Gastro-intestinal disorders: Pc 6 and St 36; TW 6 and St 36; L.I. 4 and St 36, or Pc 6 and Sp 4

6. High fever, coma, epileptic seizure: Pc 8 and Ki 1

7. Bleeding hemorrhoid: UB 54 and Lu 6

8. Laryngitis: Lu 10 and TW 2

9. Constipation: TW 6 and GB 34

10. Hemuresis: Lu 6 and TW 2

11. Insomnia: Ht 7 and Sp 6

12. Tremor in the hands: Ht 7 and L.I. 4

13. Cerebro vascular accident: L.I. 11 and GB 34

14. Mental confusion: Pc 6 and St 44

15. To clear heat and expel dampness: L.I. 4 and L.I. 11, L.I. 4 and Lu 6; Lu 11 and L.I. 1; Pc 6 and Sp 6 or Lu 10 and Ki 3

16. Itching: L.I. 11 and Sp 10 or L.I. 11 and L.I. 15

17. To regulate Qi and Blood and harmonize the interior and exterior: TW 6 and GB 34; TW 5 and GB 31 or Ki 3 or L.I. 1.

18. Alleviate swelling and pain: Ki 3 and TW 3; L.I. 4 and St 7 or L.I. 4 and St 44.

19. To facilitate breathing: Sp 9 and UB 57; Pc 6 and Ht 7 or Ki 3 and L.I. 1

20. To nourish the heart and calm the spirit: Sp 6 and Ht 7; Pc 6 and GB 31; Ki 6 and Ht 5 or Ki 3 and GB 31.

21. To expel Wind and harmonize the Liver: L.I. 4 and Liv 3; Ki 3 and Liv 3; GB 31 and St 36 or Pc 6 and St 36.

22. Uretic and edema relief: St 36 and Sp 9; Ki 6 and St 36.

E.   The Anterior-Posterior Responsive Prescribing Method

This method utilizes the points from the corresponding locations on the anterior and posterior parts of the body.

Head —

1. stroke with closed mouth: GV 26 and GV 16

2. stroke with stiff tongue: GV 15 and CV 23

3. Headache: GV 21 and GV 19

4. Nasal bleeding (epistaxis): GV 16 and L.I. 20

5. Sinusitis: UB 10 and L.I. 20

6. Mental confusion: GV19 and Yintang

Chest and Upper abdomen —

1. Chest pain or fullness: CV 17 and UB 17

2. Upper abdominal pain: CV 14 and UB 13

Lower Abdomen —

1. Lower abdominal pain: CV 6 and UB 25

2. Impotence; lumbago due to deficient kidney: CV 4 and GV 4

3. Dysmenorrhea; leukorrhea; irregular menstruation: St 28, St 29, UB 30, UB 31, UB 32, UB 33, UB 34.

Four Limbs

1. Numbness in the fingers: L.I. 3 and S.I. 3

2. Intercostal neuralgia: Pc 6 and TW 5

3. Painful wrist: Pc 6 and TW 5

4. Painful elbow joint: L.I. 11 and Ht 3

5. Painful or frozen shoulder: Jianchian and Jianho

        Jianchian: I cun above the anterior end of the axillary fold.
        Jianho: 1.5 cun above the posterior end of the axillary fold.

6. Painful hip joint: St 31 and UB 36

7. Painful knee joint: GB 34 and Sp 9

8. Painful heel or feet: Ki 2 and UB 63 or Ki 3 and UB 60

9. Ankle sprain: Ki 3 and UB 60

F. The Point Groups Alternate Prescribing Method

This method employs a different series of acupuncture points from different meridians on alternate days or weeks for treating chronic or persistent disorders.

1. Stomach or duodenal ulceration

    a. UB 20, UB 21, St 36, St 21

    b. CV 12, CV 13, St 36, UB 60, S.I. 3, S.I. 6

2. Acute or chronic gastro-enteritis

    a. Pc 6, CV 12, St 36, Pc 3 (blood letting), UB 54 (blood letting)

    b. Pc 6, CV 12, CV 13, GV 4, UB 54 (blood letting)

3. Indigestion

    a. CV 12, Sp 4, St 36 (needle and moxa)

    b. CV 12, Liv 13, St 36 (needle and moxa), Pc 6

4. Asthma

    a. UB 13, UB 15, Lu 7, L.I. 4, St 40

    b.   UB 13, GB 12, Pc 6, CV 22, Lu 5, St 40

5. Hypertension

    a.   Pc 6, L.I. 11, St 36, Yintang

    b.   Pc 6, GB 20, St 36, Liv 3

6. Insomnia

    a.   Ht 7, Pc 6, Sp 6, UB 15, St 36

    b.   Ht 7, Pc 6, Sp 1 (moxa), UB 15

7. Anemia

    a.   GV 14, UB 18, Pc 6, St 36, UB 65

    b.   GV 14, UB 17, GV 4, St 36, Sp 9

8. Sciatica

    a.   GB 30, GB 31, UB 25, UB 36, UB 54, UB 60

    b.   GB 30, GB 34, UB 36, UB 54, UB 60

9. Facial Paralysis (Bell's Palsy)

    a.   Taiyang, St 6, St 7, L.I. 4

    b.   Taiyang, St 7, L.I. 20, GB 20

10. Nocturnal enuresis (wetting bed)

    a.   CV 3, CV 4, Sp 6, UB 23

    b.   CV 3, Sp 6, Sp 9, UB 23

11. Dysmenorrhea

  a. CV 3, CV 4, Sp 6, St 36

  b. CV 3, CV 6, Sp 6, Sp 10, Ki 3

12. Infertility

  a. Pc 6, CV 4, Sp 6 (needle and moxa), GV 4, UB 23

  b. CV 3, CV 4, St 36, Sp 6 (needle and moxa), GV 4, UB 23

13. Glaucoma

  a. GB 20, Taiyang, L.I. 4, UB 1

  b. GB 20, Taiyang, L.I. 4, Yuyao

14. Sinusitis

  a. L.I. 20, L.I. 4, Yintang

  b. L.I. 20, St 36, Yintang

15. Diabetes

  a. CV 4, CV 12, UB 23, Sp 6 (needle and moxa), Ki 3 (needle and moxa)

  b. CV 4, CV 6, UB 23 (needle and moxa), Ki 7

16. Constipation

  a. TW 5, GB 34, Sp 3, Ki 6

  b. TW 5, GB 34, Sp 3, UB 54

G. The External-Internal Related Meridian Prescribing Method

This method involves the use of points from two meridians that are indicated by the symptoms of their respective externally-internally related meridians.

The following is the pattern of externally-internally related meridians:

Taiyin	Lu <———>	L.I.	Yangming
	Sp <———>	St	
Shaoyin	Ht <———>	S.I.	Taiyang
	Ki <———>	UB	
Jueyin	Pc <———>	TW	Shaoyang
	Liv <———>	GB	

1. **Lu <———> L.I.**

   Lu 5 and L.I. 4 : cough
   Lu 3 and L.I. 4 : nasal bleeding

2. **Sp <———> St**

   Sp 4 and St 36: gastro-intestinal disorders
   Sp 10, Sp 6 and St 28, St 29: irregular menstruation
   Sp 1 and St 45: nightmares

3. **Ht <———> S.I.**

   Ht 7 and S.I. 3: sedative function for organs as well as pain relief
   Ht 6 and S.I. 3: night sweating

4. **Ki <———> UB**

   Ki 3 and UB 2: insomnia
   Ki 3 and UB 13, UB 15: mental confusion

5. Pc <———> TW

   Pc 6 and TW 2: fatigue
   Pc 6 and TW 5 : tendonitis (arms)

6. Liv<———> GB

   Liv 3 and GB 31: anxiety, anger
   Liv 13 and GB 31: intercostal neuralgia

H. The Six Conductions Prescribing Method

Based on the principle of the Yin-Yang Tai-Chi figure below, this method helps to regulate, tonify and disperse Qi and Blood at the same time.

The following drawing describes the six conductions in the Yin-Yang Tai-Chi figure. (It is different from the exterior-interior relation of the Zang-Fu organs).

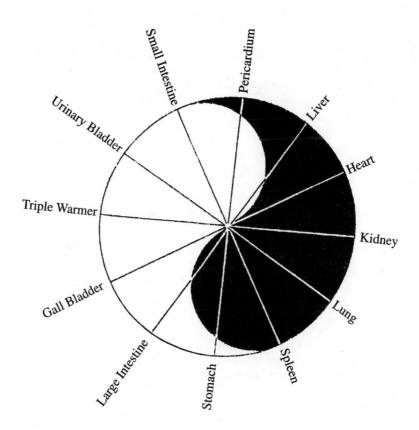

Taiyin   Lu <———> UB   Taiyang

              Sp <———> S.I.

Shaoyin   Ht <———> GB   Shaoyang

              Ki <———> TW

Jueyin   Pc <———> St   Yangming

              Liv <———> L.I.

The Six Conductions in the Yin-Yang Tai-Chi figures was mentioned in the book, *Basic Conceptions to Chinese Medicine,* dating from the Ming Dynasty (A.D. 1368-1644). This theory is applied not only in the treatment of pain disorders but also in treating disorders of the internal organs.

1. For pain relief:

    a. Lu 5: pain along the Urinary Bladder meridian

    b. Ht 7: pain along the Gall Bladder meridian

    c. Pc 6: pain along the Stomach meridian

    d. TW 5: pain along the Kidney meridian

    e. L.I. 4: pain along the Liver meridian

    f. S.I. 4: pain along the Spleen meridian

2. For disorders of the internal organs:

    a. Lu <———> UB

        Lung diseases: disperse UB points (blood letting at UB 54)
        Urinary bladder disorders: clear Lung Qi (disperse Lu points)

b. Sp <————> S.I.

Spleen conditions: disperse S.I. fire
Small Intestine disharmonies: tonify Spleen

c. Ht <————> GB

Heart conditions: disperse GB points
Gall Bladder disorders: tonify Ht points

d. Ki <————> TW

Kidney problems: disperse TW points
Triple Warmer disharmonies: tonify Ki points

e. Pc <————> St

Pericardium disorders: tonify St points
Stomach conditions: disperse Pc points

f. Liv<————> L.I.

Liver diseases: disperse L.I. points
Large Intestine problems: both tonify and disperse Liver Qi

I. The Following Meridian Prescribing Method

This technique employs acupuncture points from specific meridians
whose pathways correspond to the location of the disease. This method
is usually associated with the "Move Qi" method and the needles are
usually inserted in the healthy side of the body (see Part III: technique).

1. If the disorder is located on the internal aspect of the arm
    and chest region, select points from the three Yin merid-
    ians of the hands.

2. When the problem is located at the internal-lateral aspect
    of the feet, chest and abdominal regions, select points from
    the three Yin meridians of the feet.

3. If a condition is located on the external side of the arm or the head and facial regions, choose points from the three Yang meridians of the hands.

4. When a disease is located at the external-lateral aspect of the head, trunk, abdominal or back regions, select points from the three Yang meridians of the feet.

The following is an outline of the relationship between the location of disease and prescribing and combining points:

Location of Disease	Belongs to Meridians	Major Points	Combining Points
HEAD:			
Posterior	UB	UB 60, UB 65	GB20, GV16
Lateral	GB, TW	GB 39, TW 3	St 8
Parietal	GV, UB, Liv	UB 65, Liv 3	GV 20
Frontal	St	St 44	St 41
Five Sense Organs	St, S.I., CV	St 44, S.I. 3	L.I. 20, S.I. 6, S.I. 7, CV 24
NECK and SHOULDER:			
Posterior	GB, GV, UB	UB 60, GV 16	GB 20, S.I. 11
Lateral	L.I. , S.I., TW	L.I. 4, S.I. 3, TW 5	Lu 7, S.I. 11
Frontal	St, CV	St 41, CV 22	Lu 7

Back & Lumbar	UB, GV, S.I.	UB 60, UB 54, SI3	GV14, GV4 GB 34, UB 23

Chest, Hypochondriac & Costal Regions	CV, GV, PC GB, Ki, St SP, Liv	GB 38, CV 17 Ki 3, St 40, Liv 3	TW 6

Abdominal Region	CV, GB, Liv Sp	CV 12, CV 4, Sp 6, Liv 3 GB 34	St 36, CV 3, Liv 13

UPPER ARMS:

Internal	Lu, Pc, Ht	Liv 3, Lu 9, Pc 8, Ht 5	Lu 5, Pc 3,
External	L.I. , TW, S.I	L.I. 4, TW 5, S.I. 3	L.I. 11,TW 10, S.I. 8

LOWER LIMBS:

Anterior	St	St 36	St 40
Posterior	UB	UB 54	GB 30, UB 36
Internal	Liv, Sp, Ki	Sp 6, Liv 3, Ki 3	Liv 14
External	GB	GB 34	GB 30,UB 65

J. The Connected Meridian Prescribing Method

This technique utilizes points from meridians that are connected to each other. This method is usually associated with the "Move Qi" or "Tractive Method" of acupuncture techniques (see Part III) that are used to enhance the therapeutic effect. Points are selected from the remote parts of the body and needled in the healthy side of the body with gentle massage applied to the area of disorder both before and after needle manipulation.

The following describes the pattern of the Connected Meridian among the twelve meridians:

Meridians: **Meridians:**

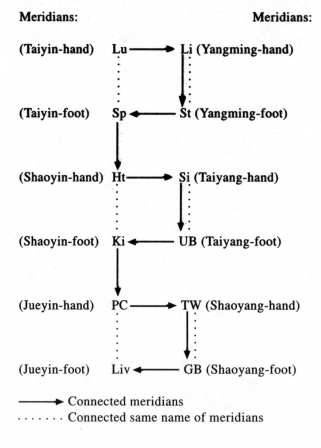

(Taiyin-hand)	Lu ──→ Li (Yangming-hand)
(Taiyin-foot)	Sp ◄── St (Yangming-foot)
(Shaoyin-hand)	Ht ──→ Si (Taiyang-hand)
(Shaoyin-foot)	Ki ◄── UB (Taiyang-foot)
(Jueyin-hand)	PC ──→ TW (Shaoyang-hand)
(Jueyin-foot)	Liv ◄── GB (Shaoyang-foot)

──→ Connected meridians
· · · · · · · Connected same name of meridians

The practitioner should diagnose the main syndrome and determine which meridian is associated with it and apply this method to select a prescription. Selection is from among the Five-Shu points, the Xi (Cleft) points or the Luo (Connecting) points of connected meridians. For example, sciatica belongs to the GB meridian, and the TW meridian is connected to the GB; thus, TW 6 and GB 30 are chosen for sciatica. Similarly, Pc 7 and Ki 3 are chosen for pain in the heel, while Sp 4 and St 34 are chosen for stomachache.

The following are the diseases treated by the connected meridian prescribing method:

Name of Disease	Belongs to Meridian	Connected Meridian	Select Point
Pharyngeal Pain	Lu	Lower Connect to L.I.	L.I. 4
Toothache	St	Upper Connect to L.I.	L.I.4
Insomnia	Ht	Upper Connect to Sp	Sp 6
Stomachache	St	Lower Connect to Sp	Sp 4
Dizziness	Liv	Upper Connect to GB	GB38
Abdominal Pain	Sp	Upper Connect to St	St 36

Shoulder Pain	L.I.	Lower Connect to St	St 38
	S.I.	Lower Connect to UB	UB 57
	TW	Lower Connect to GB	GB 34

Lower Limb Pain	St	Upper Connect to L.I.	L.I. 7
	UB	Upper Connect to S.I.	S.I. 4
	St	Upper Connect to L.I.	L.I. 10
	GB	Upper Connect to TW	TW 5
	UB	Upper Connect to S.I.	S.I. 3

Lumbar Pain	Ki	Upper Connect to UB	UB 54

Heel Pain	Ki	Lower Connect to Pc	Pc 7

Intercostal Neuralgia	GB	Upper Connect to TW	TW 6

K. Point Prescription Using the Through Meridian Method

This method of point selection is based on the use of points from the three Yin and the three Yang meridians of the hands and feet. This method is associated with the Move Qi method in acupuncture technique (see Part Three) and is usually applied in the treatment of disorders which are located in a specific region the associated meridian/s. The following table shows the connection between the associated meridians.

3 Yin Meridians of hands	Connection place or point	3 Yin meridians of feet
Taiyin (Lu)	Lu 1	Taiyin (Sp)
Shaoyin (Ht)	Central heart	Shaoyin (Ki)
Jueyin (Pc)	Pc 1	Jueyin (Liv)

3 Yang meridians of hands		3 Yang meridians of feet
Taiyang (S.I.)	UB 1	Taiyang (UB)
Shaoyang (TW)	GB 1	Shaoyang (GB)
Yangming (L.I.)	L.I. 20	Yangming (St)

The following is an outline of the disease location and point selection according to the Through Meridian prescribing method.

Location of disease	Belongs to meridian	Selecting point	Belongs to meridian
L.I. 5	Yangming-hand	St 41	Yangming-foot
S.I. 5	Taiyang-hand	UB 60	Taiyang-foot
TW 4	Shaoyang-hand	GB 40	Shaoyang-foot
Lu 10	Taiyin-hand	Sp 4	Taiyin-foot
Ht 7	Shaoyin-hand	Ki 3	Shaoyin-foot

Pc 7	Jueyin-hand	Liv 4	Jueyin-foot
St 43	Yangming-foot	L.I. 4	Yangming-hand
UB 65	Taiyang-foot	S.I. 3	Taiyang-hand
GB 41	Shaoyang-foot	Tw 3	Shaoyang-hand
Sp 9	Taiyin-foot	Lu 5	Taiyin-hand
Ki 10	Shaoyin-foot	Ht 3	Shaoyin-hand
Liv 5	Jueyin-foot	Pc 4	Jueyin-hand

The point prescription based on the Through Meridian prescribing method is selected from the corresponding point of one or both sides of the meridian of the same name. For example, St 41 (Yangming) is chosen for treating pain located in L.I. 5 area (Yangming); S.I. 7 (Taiyang) is chosen for treating pain in the UB 57 area (Taiyang). Therefore, this method is generally used for treating diseases which are located in the four limbs.

L.   The Applied Prescribing Method of Five-Shu Points

The Five-Shu Points Method of point selection is based on the specific actions of the Five-Shu points which are distributed below the elbow and knee joints of upper and lower limbs. Those five specific points are the Jing-Well, Rong-Spring, Shu-Stream , Jing-River and Her-Sea. Their respective therapeutic properties are as follows: Jing-Well points are indicated in mental illness and chest fullness; Rong-Spring Points in febrile disease; Shu-Stream Points in Bi-syndrome; Jing-River Points in asthma, cough, and cold and heat syndromes; and Her-Sea Points in diarrhea. The following is the interpretation of indications of the Five-Shu Points:

    1.   Jing-Well Points:

        The Jing-Well points are associated with the Yin organs and are related to the Wood element. The Yin organ of

Wood is the liver. When the Liver Qi stagnates or becomes constrained, the Middle Warmer and the Upper Warmer can become affected and chest fullness can result. Liver Qi stagnation can be due to mental problems; thus the symptoms of mental illness and chest fullness can be related to the Wood element and the associated Yin organ, the liver.

2.   Rong-Spring Points:

This group of points is related to the element of Fire and to the Yin organ of the heart. The heart dominates the Blood which nourishes the whole body. When the body is attacked by an exogenous pathogenic factor, the blood circulation is impaired and, as a result of the disharmony of the internal organs, internal heat is generated. Rong-Spring points are used to treat febrile diseases and are associated with the Fire element.

3   Shu-Stream Points:

Shu-Stream points are related to the Earth element and to the spleen. When the spleen loses its normal function of transformation and transportation, a condition of accumulation and dampness with phlegm results. This dampness, especially in combination with Cold, can affect all areas of the body, but especially the joints, causing Bi-syndrome. The Shu-Stream points are selected in the treatment of Bi-syndrome.

4.   Jing-River Points:

Jing-River Points are related to the element of Metal and to the lung. The lung dominates the skin and hair as well as the functions of respiration and body temperature. The lung is easily affected by invasion of exogenous pathogenic Wind or Cold which results in the retention of damp-phlegm or phlegm-heat in the lung. The lung looses its function of descending or ascending the Qi giving rise to cough and asthma as well as Cold and Heat syndromes. These conditions are treated by using the Jing-River Points.

5. Her-Sea Points:

The Her-Sea points are related to the Water element and to
the organ of the kidneys. If the kidney and bladder lose
their ability to control water metabolism, the excess water
with pathogenic heat remains in the urinary bladder and
affects both the digestive system and the intestines. The
Her-Sea points are useful for treating diarrhea and other
intestinal disorders.

The following is a table of the Five-Shu Points of the twelve meridians:

Five-Shu Points:	Jing Well	Rong Spring	Shu Stream	Jing River	Her Sea
Five Elements:	Wood	Fire	Earth	Metal	Water
Specific Effect:	A	B	C	D	E

Yin Meridians

Lu (Hand)-Taiyin	Lu 11	Lu 10	Lu 9	Lu 8	Lu 5
Ht (Hand)-Shaoyin	Ht 9	Ht 8	Ht 7	Ht 4	Ht 3
Pc (Hand)-Jueyin	Pc 9	Pc 8	Pc 7	Pc 5	Pc 3
Sp (Foot)-Taiyin	Sp 1	Sp 2	Sp 3	Sp 5	Sp 9
Ki (Foot)-Shaoyin	Ki 1	Ki 2	Ki 3	Ki 7	Ki 10
Liv (Foot)Jueyin	Liv 1	Liv 2	Liv 3	Liv 4	Liv 8
Five Elements:	Metal	Water	Wood	Fire	Earth
Specific Effect:	A	B	C	D	E

Yang Meridians

L.I. (Hand)-Yangming	L.I. 1	L.I. 2	L.I. 3	L.I. 5	L.I.11
S.I. (Hand)-Taiyang	S.I. 1	S.I. 2	S.I. 3	S.I. 5	S.I. 18
TW (Hand)-Shaoyang	TW 1	TW 2	TW 3	TW 6	TW 10
ST (Foot)-Yangming	St 45	St 44	St 43	St 41	St 36
UB (Foot)-Taiyang	UB 67	UB 66	UB 65	UB 60	UB 40
GB (Foot)-Shaoyang	GB 44	GB 43	GB 41	GB 38	GB 34

A. mental illness, chest fullness B. febrile disease C. Bi-syndrome
D. asthma, cough, Cold and Heat syndromes E. diarrhea and intestinal disorders

The indications and specific functions of the Five-Shu Points are as follows:

1. Jing-Well Points

    a. the onset of various disorders: excess syndromes (blood letting); deficient syndromes (moxibustion)

    b. internal organ dysfunction: Sp 1 (moxibustion), Liv 1 (moxibustion)

    c. coma: Liv 1

    d. difficult labor: UB 67 (moxibustion)

    e. uterine hemorrhage or polymenorrhea: L.I. 1 (moxibustion)

    f. pharyngeal pain or swelling, pharyngitis and tonsillitis: Lu 11 (blood letting)

    g. mental depression: Ki 1 (moxibustion)

    h. anger: GB 44 (bloodletting)

    i. hiccough: Ht 9

    j. chest pain or fullness: Ht 9

2. Rong-Spring Points

    a. acute bronchitis: Lu 10 (blood letting), L.I. 2 (blood letting)

    b. various febrile disorders: Lu 10 (blood letting)

    c. intercostal neuralgia: Liv 10 (blood letting)

3. Shu-Stream Points

    a. various chronic disorders: needle bilaterally with moxibustion

b. chronic joint pain in the upper limbs due to Bi-syndrome (arthritis): Lu 9, Pc 7

c. chronic joint pain in the lower limbs due to Bi-syndrome (arthritis): Liv 3, Ki 3

d. intermittent heat and cold syndrome: S.I. 3

4. Jing-River Points

a. various disorders which attack any organ: needle bilaterally with moxibustion or blood letting

b. asthma due to Deficiency of Lung or Kidney: Lu 8, Ki 7

c. cough: Lu 8

d. clenched mouth due to cerebro-vascular accident: Sp 5

5. Her-Sea Points

a. adjust physiological function of the Fu (hollow) organs: needle bilaterally with moxibustion

b. abdominal distention: St 36

c. asthma resulting in stagnation of the Middle Jiao: Lu 5

d. diarrhea: GB 34

e. indigestion: L.I. 11, St 36

f. to improve digestion, respiration and metabolism: L.I. 11, St 36

M. The Applied Prescribing Method of Mother and Son Points

In this method, points from the Five-Shu Points of the original meridian, or hetero-meridian, are selected according to the relationship
of inter-promotion and inter-action among the five elements to enhance tonification and dispersion. This method is usually applied to
treat disorders of the internal organs, but can also be applied in disorders of the channels and collaterals. Before this method of prescription selection is applied, a number of factors have to be considered:
the nature of the disease (excessive or deficient syndromes), the relationship between the internal organs and the five elements, the action
and location of the Five-Shu Points, and the principles of tonifying
the mother point for deficient syndromes and dispersing the son point
for excessive syndromes. The relationships of inter-promoting and
inter-acting among the five elements is pictured in the following diagram. This is commonly called the creative and control cycles:

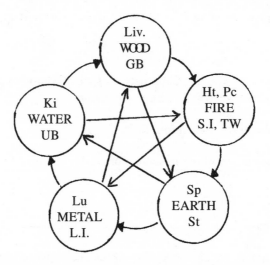

Based on the above chart, Metal promotes Water, Water promotes
Wood, Wood promotes Fire, Fire promotes Earth and Earth promotes
Metal. Lu and L.I. belong to Metal, Ki and UB belong to Water, Liv
and GB belong to Wood, Ht and S.I. belong to Fire (emperor Fire),
Pc and TW belong to Fire (minister Fire) and Sp and St belong to
Earth. The promoting element is thought of as the "mother" and the
promoted element as the "son". The mother and son points for
tonification and dispersion are on pages 170 and 171.

Based on the following table, for a patient with a Deficient Kidney syndrome, Ki 7 will be chosen for tonification because the Kidney belongs to the Water element and Water is promoted by Metal. Therefore, the Metal (mother) point of the original meridian is selected (Homo-meridian selection). Also for tonification is the point Lu 8, the mother point of the mother meridian (Hetero-meridian selection).

In a syndrome of Kidney Excess such as a feverish sensation in the palms and soles and night sweating due to insufficiency of Kidney Yin, the Wood point (Ki 1) from the original meridian (Homo-meridian selection) and Liv 1 from the succeeding meridian are used for dispersing the excess (Hetero-meridian selection). These points are chosen based on the mother and son applied prescribing method.

Disorders relating to the other organs listed in the table on the following two pages follow the same examples above.

The Mother and Son Points for Tonification and Dispersion

TONIFICATION

Solid & Hollow Organs	Original Meridians (Five Elements)	Promoting Elements	Mother Points	Mother Meridians	Mother Points
Gall bladder	Wood	Water	Hsia Hsi (GB 43)	Urinary bladder	Tung Ku (UB 66)
Liver	Wood	Water	Chu Chuan (Liv 8)	Kidney	Ying Ku (Ki 10)
Small intestine	Fire	Wood	Hou Hsi (S.I. 3)	Gall bladder	Lin Chih (GB 41)
Heart	Fire	Wood	Shao Chung (HL 9)	Liver	Ta Tun (Liv 1)
Stomach	Earth	Fire	Chieh Tsi (St 41)	Small intestine	Yang Ku (S.I. 5)
Spleen	Earth	Fire	Da Du (Sp 2)	Heart	Shao Fu (Ht 8)
Large intestine	Metal	Earth	Chu Chih (L.I. 11)	Stomach	Tsu San L.I. (St 36)
Lung	Metal	Earth	Tai Yuan (Lu 9)	Spleen	Tai Pai (Sp 3)
Urinary bladder	Water	Metal	Chi Yin (UB 67)	Large intestine	Shang Yang (L.I. 1)
Kidney	Water	Metal	Fu Liu (Ki 7)	Lung	Ching Chu (Lu 8)
Triple Warmer	Fire	Wood	Chung Tu (TW 3)	Gall bladder	Lin Chih (GB 41)
Pericardium	Fire	Wood	Chong Chung (Pc 9)	Liver	Ta Tun (Liv 1)

DISPERSION

Solid & Hollow Organs	Original Meridians (Five Elements)	Promoted Elements	Son Points	Son Meridians	Son Points
Gall bladder	Wood	Fire	Yang Pu (GB 38)	Small intestine	Yang Ku (S.I. 5)
Liver	Wood	Fire	Hsing Chien (Liv 2)	Heart	Shao Fu (Ht 8)
Small intestine	Fire	Earth	Hsiao Hai (Si 8)	Stomach	Thsu San L.I. (St 36)
Heart	Fire	Earth	Shen men (Ht 7)	Spleen	Tai Pai (Sp 3)
Stomach	Earth	Metal	Li Tui (St 45)	Large intestine	Shang Yang (L.I. 1)
Spleen	Earth	Metal	Shang Chiu (Sp 5)	Lung	Ching Chu (Lu 8)
Large intestine	Metal	Water	Erh Chien (L.I. 2)	Urinary bladder	Tung Ku (UB 66)
Lung	Metal	Water	Chih Tseh (Lu 5)	Kidney	Ying Ku (Ki 10)
Urinary bladder	Water	Wood	Shu Ku (UB 65)	Gall bladder	Lin Chih (GB 41)
Kidney	Water	Wood	Yung Chuan (Ki 1)	Liver	Ta Tun (Liv 1)
Triple Warmer	Fire	Earth	Tiem Ching (TW 10)	Stomach	Tsu San Li (St 36)
Pericardium	Fire	Earth	Ta Ling (Pc 7)	Spleen	Tai Pai (Sp 3)

N. The Applied Prescribing Method of The Three Parts.

In this technique, points are chosen from among local, adjacent and remote points according to the distribution of points, their indications and the direction, or course, of the meridians. It is also called "the sky-earth-people prescribing method," and it is comprehensively used in acupuncture prescriptions. The chart below demonstrates how the three parts prescribing method is applied to treat common disorders.

Symptoms	Local Points	Adjacent Points	Remote Points
Coma	GV 20	GV 26	Ki 1
Tinnitus due to Kidney Deficiency	S.I.19	UB 23	St 36
Difficulty hearing due to damp heat retained in the gall bladder	TW 21	GB 43	Tw 5
Nasal Congestion or nose bleeding	L.I. 20	GV 23	L.I. 4
Pharyngitis	L.I. 4 or TW 2	L.I. 11 Lu 10	Liv 3 Liv 3
Abdominal pain or stomachache	CV 12	St 25 Pc 6	St 36
Headache	Yintang Taiyang	GV 23	GB 31 SP 4

Dizziness	Taiyang	GB 20	CV 4 Sp 6 St 36 Ki 3
Insomnia	Yintang	GV 20	Ht 7 Pc 6 Sp 6 Ki 3 Sp 4
Diarrhea	St 25	CV 12	St 36 CV 6 L.I. 4 Sp 4
Lumbago or lower back pain	UB 23	GB 30 GV 4	UB 54
Nocturnal enuresis	CV 3	CV 4	Sp 6 Liv 1
Impotence	CV 3	CV 4	Sp 6 Ht 7 Sp 4 Ki 3
Amenorrhea	CV 3	CV 4	Sp 6 Sp 10
Dysmenorrhea	CV 3	CV 4	Sp 6 Sp 10 L.I. 4 St 36 GB 31 Liv 3

Neck Stiffness	GB 20	S.I. 3	GB 39

O. The Applied Prescribing Method of Shu-Mu Points

This method utilizes points from among the Back-Shu points and their corresponding points of CV, Lu, Liv, St and GB meridians. Shu points are located on the UB meridian: they are a Qi import place from the internal organs to the back of body. Mu points are located on the CV, Lu, Liv, St and GB meridians: they are a Qi accumulating place from the internal organs to the chest and abdominal regions. Whenever pathological changes occur in the internal organs, there is often a reaction spot or tender spot at the corresponding Back-Shu Point, or at the corresponding Front-Mu Point.

The Back-Shu Points and the Front-Mu Points can be used separately or in combination. For example, stomachache with vomiting is treated by CV 12 or CV 12 and UB 21, and by Lu 1 or Lu 1 and UB 13 for cough. The Back-Shu Points also can be used in treating disorders of the sense organs that are related to their corresponding internal organs. For example, UB 15, the Back-Shu Point of the heart, may be chosen to treat sores on the tip of tongue since the heart opens into the tongue. Similarly, UB 23 is chosen for the treatment of tinnitus because the kidney opens into the ear. Clinically, the therapeutic pattern of the Shu-Mu Points applied prescribing method follows certain rules:

1. for disorders of the kidney, heart, lung, liver and spleen: Back-Shu Points

2. for disorders of the stomach, urinary bladder, gall bladder, large intestine, small intestine and sanjiao (chest, epigastrium, and hypogastrium): Front-Mu Points

3. for acute disorders: Front-Mu Points

4. chronic disorders: Back-Shu Points

5. excessive syndromes: Front-Mu Points

6. deficient syndromes: Back-Shu Points

The following table shows the indications of Shu-Mu Points:

The Indications of Shu-Mu Points

Internal Organs	Shu-Points/Mu-Points	Indications
Lung	UB 13/Lu 1	respiratory diseases: cough, asthma, chest fullness
Pericardium	UB 14/CV 17	heart diseases: tachycardia, pain in the heart
Heart	UB 15/CV 14	heart and stomach diseases: tachycardia palpitations, stomach-ache
Liver	UB 18/Liv 14	liver and stomach diseases: pain
Gall bladder	UB 19/GB 24	liver and gall bladder diseases: jaundice and intercostal neuralgia
Spleen	UB 20/Liv 13	liver and spleen diseases: abdominal distention, abdominal pain, enlarged spleen or liver and indigestion

Stomach	UB 21/CV 12	stomach diseases: stomachache distention and poor appetite
Triple Warmer	UB 22/CV 5	dysfunction of fluid metabolism: edema, ascites and diarrhea
Kidney	UB 23/GB 25	kidney and genital organs diseases: lumbago impotence, emission and soreness of lower back
Large Intestine	UB 25/St 25	intestinal diseases: constipation, diarrhea and abdominal pain
Small Intestine	UB 27/CV 4	small intestine, urinary bladder and genital organ disorders
Urinary Bladder	UB 28/CV 3	urinary bladder and genital organ disorders: incontinence of urine, oligurea, polyurea, irregular menstruation and emission

P. Applied Prescribing Method of Yuan (Source)-Luo (Connecting) Points

This method involves the use of points located in the areas of the wrists and ankles for treating the associated internal organs and the use of points located on the connected place of external-internal related meridians. Clinically, these two groups of points can be used in conjunction with each other or separately. Needles inserted at the Yuan Points will open the Sanjiao (chest, upper and lower abdominal areas) and adjust the physiological function of internal organs. For example, Lu 9 is used in the treatment of lung diseases; Liv 3 for treating liver diseases. Selecting the Luo points will treat syndromes of the respective external-internal related meridians. For example, Sp 4 for the treatment of diseases of the spleen and stomach, as the spleen and stomach are external-internal related meridians. Other external-internal related meridians are: Lu/L.I. meridians; Ki/UB meridians; Ht/S.I. meridians; Pc/ TW meridians; and Liv/GB meridians. The coordination of the Yuan-Luo Points in the prescription will enhance the therapeutic effect.

In general, it is best to choose the Yuan point of the affected meridian and combine it with the Luo point of its external-internal related meridian. An example of this would be the use of Ki 3 (Yuan point) for treating kidney diseases in conjunction with UB 58 (Luo Point) to enhance the effect of treatment.

It is very effective to apply Luo Points in blood letting to treat many kinds of excessive syndromes. The following are prescriptions for the use of the Luo points with blood letting among the twelve meridians for treating various excessive syndromes:

1. Lu 7: heat in the palms of both hands

2. Ht 5: burning sensation in the heart

3. Pc 6: pain in the heart region.

4. S.I. 7: painful elbow joint

5. L.I. 6: toothache and deafness

6. TW 5: spasm of the elbow muscle and tendon

7. UB 58: back pain

8. St 40: epilepsy

9. GB 37: internal heat retention

10. Sp 4: intestinal pain

11. Ki 4: hemmorrhoid

12. Liv 5: swollen testicle(s) and hernia

13. GV 1: back muscle spasm and tightness

14. CV 15: acute abdominal pain

The table below lists the indications of Yuan-Luo Points:

The Indications of Yuan-Luo Points

Location of disease	Yuan-Luo Points	Indications
Lu/L.I.	Lu 9/L.I. 6	Trachitis; pharyngitis; shortness of breath; excessive sputum; heat in palms of hands; pain in both breasts; shoulder pain
L.I./Lu	L.I. 4/Lu 7	toothache, gingivitis; runny nose, shoulder pain

Sp/St	Sp 3/St 40	abdominal pain; vomiting; constipation; jaundice; leg pain
St/Sp	St 42/Sp 4	Nasal bleeding; facial paralysis; abdominal distention; leg pain
Ht/S.I.	Ht 7/S.I. 7	tachycardia; upper limb pain; chest pain
S.I./Ht	S.I. 4/Ht 5	shoulder pain; neck stiffness; deafness; upper limb pain
Ki/UB	Ki 3/UB 58	fatigue; no appetite; dimness of vision; low back pain, leg weakness or pain
UB/Ki	UB 64/Ki 4	neck stiffness or pain; low back pain; leg pain; epilepsy; eye disease; hemorrhoid

TW/Pc	TW 4/Pc 6	deafness; pharyngitis; conjunctivitis shoulder pain; back pain; constipation; urinary disorder
Pc/TW	Pc 7/TW 5	finger spasm; chest pain; wrist pain; tendonitis in the arms; anxiety; heat in the palms; mental disorder
Liv/GB	Liv 3/GB 37	testitis; hernia; vomiting; chest pain; diarrhea; abdominal pain; incontinence of urine; oligurea
GB/Liv	GB 40/Liv 5	chest pain; intercostal neuralgia; headache; goiter; eye disorder

Q. The Applied Prescribing Method of Xi (Cleft) Points

With the use of this prescription method, the Xi Cleft points are chosen for treating acute disorders which occur in their respective related organs. Xi Cleft points are places where the Qi accumulates
along the twelve meridians and the four extraordinary vessels (Yinwei,
Yangwei, Yinchiao and Yangchiao). Lu 6, the Xi point of lung meridian, is chosen for lung related hemoptysis; Ht 6 or Pc 4 is selected for
angina; St 34 is used for stomachache; and GB 35 applied for painful
due to gall stones.

Clinically, Xi Cleft points and the eight influential points are combined in prescriptions for more effective results. For example, Lu 6

and CV 17 are chosen for treating asthma associated with bronchitis, while St 34 and CV 12 are needled for stomach spasm. The following is the table of the Xi (Cleft) points of the twelve meridians and the extraordinary vessels:

Meridians of the hands and their Xi points	Meridians of the feet and their Xi points	Extra Meridians and their Xi points
Lu: Lu 6	Sp: Sp 8	Yinwei: Ki 9
Ht: Ht 6	Ki: Ki 5	Yangwei: GB 35
Pc: Pc 4	Liv: Liv 6	Yinchiao: Ki 8
L.I.: L.I. 7	St: St 34	Yangchiao:UB59
S.I.: S.I. 6:	UB: UB 63	
TW: TW 7	GB: GB 36	

Indications of the Xi (Cleft) Points

1. Lu 6: cough, headache; sore throat; angina

2. Ht 6: night sweat; angina

3. Pc 4: painful chest or heart area; nose bleeding; hemoptysis

4. L.I. 7: swelling of the face, angina, sore throat

5. S.I. 6: pain, swelling or twitching of the hands and arms; dimness of vision

6. TW 7: soreness and numbness of the hands and arms

7. Sp 8: abdominal distention; intercostal neuralgia; retention of urine; acute edema; irregular menstruation

8. Ki 5:   chest fullness or pain; painful feet or heels

9. Liv 6: lower abdominal pain; hernia; uterine bleeding

10. St 34: stomachache; painful breast; painful knee

11. UB 63: epilepsy; deafness

12. GB 36: headache; neck stiffness

13. GB 35: painful knee and weakness of feet or legs

14. Ki 9:   hysteria; epilepsy

15. UB 59: headache; mental illness

16. Ki 8:   irregular menstruation; uterine bleeding; testitis

R. The Applied Prescribing Method of Eight Influential Points

This prescription method employs points which are located at the Qi meeting places of their respective tissues or organs in order to treat associated disorders. Clinically, the eight influential points are often combined in prescriptions with the Xi (Cleft) points for treating acute disorders, febrile disorders, painful and inflammatory disorders.

One common use of the applied prescribing method of the eight influential points is the use of CV 7 and Lu 6 in the treatment of asthma associated with cough or bronchitis. Other examples are: CV 12 and St 34 for stomachache; Lu 9 and Ht 6 for varix or vasculitis; CV 17 and Lu 6 for cough with bloody sputum; Liv 13 and Ki 5 for nephritis with fever; and GB 34 and TW 7 for tendonitis in the arms.

The following table lists the influential points and their respective tissue or organ:

Tissue or Organ	Influential Point
Zang organs (solid organs)	Liv 13
Fu organs (hollow organs)	CV 12
Qi (respiratory system)	CV 17
Blood	UB 17
Tendons	GB 34
Pulse, Blood vessels	Lu 9
Bone	UB 11
Marrow	GB 39

Generally speaking, the following guidelines are applicable:

1. Liv 13: for treating disorders of the five solid organs, but particularly for treating disorders of the liver and spleen

2. CV 12: for treating disorders of the six hollow organs, but primarily for treating disorders of the stomach and large intestines

3. CV17: for treating all kinds of Qi disorders, e.g. chest fullness, shortness of breath, hiccough and asthma

4. UB 17: for treating all kinds of blood disorders, e.g. hematuria, hemoptysis, nose bleeding, cough with bloody sputum, bloody stool, hemorrhoidal bleeding, and hematoma and hemorrhage due to physical injuries

5. GB 34: for treating tendon problems, e.g. muscular atrophy, spasm, pain, and stiffness and weakness of the joints including hemiplegia

6. Lu 9: for treating pulse and blood vessel disorders, e.g. disorders
    of the heart and lung; weakness of the pulse; deficiency of both
    Qi and Blood

7. UB 11: for treating bone disorders, e.g. arthritis; painful joints;
    osteitis

8. GB 39: for treating disorders of the bone marrow, e.g. paralysis
    and CVA (cerebral vascular accident)

S. The Applied Prescribing Method of Eight Confluent Points

This prescription method employs points which are located at the
exchange places of the twelve regular meridians and the eight extra
meridians. They are used for treating disorders of the extra meridians
and their related Zang/Fu meridians. Four of the eight confluent points
are located on the upper extremities and the other four are situated on
the lower extremities. Clinically, if an extra meridian is affected, the
point of its related Zang/Fu meridian is chosen. For example, if the
Yinwei meridian is affected Pc 6 may be chosen. Furthermore, points
of the upper extremities may be combined with their coupled points
on the lower extremities and vice versa. For example, Pc 6 and Sp 4
are chosen for treating disorders of the heart, chest and stomach. The
table below lists the eight confluent points and their indications.

Eight Confluent Points	Regular Meridian	Extra Meridian	Indications
Pc 6	Pc	Yinwei	disorders of the heart,
Sp 4	Sp	Chong	chest and stomach
S.I. 3	S.I.	Du	disorders of the neck,
UB 62	UB	Yangchiao	shoulder, back and inner canthus

| TW 5 | TW | Yangwei | disorders of the |
| GB 41 | GB | Dai | retroauricle, cheek and outer canthus |

| Lu 7 | Lu | Ren | disorders of the throat, |
| Ki 6 | Ki | Yinchiao | chest and lung |

1. Pc 6 (penetrates the Yinwei) and Sp 4 (penetrates the Chong): disorders of the heart, stomach and chest.

2. S.I. 3 (penetrates the Du) and UB 62 (penetrates the Yangchiao): disorders of the head, neck, ear, shoulder, small intestine and urinary bladder.

3. GB 41 (penetrates the Dai) and TW 5 (penetrates the Yangwei): disorders of the eye, ear, facial and neck regions.

4. Lu 7 (penetrates the Ren) and Ki 6 (penetrates the Yinchaio): disorder of the throat, chest and lung.

T. The Applied Prescribing Method of Original Meridian

Here, to enhance the therapeutic needling effect, the acupuncturist employs one or more points from the meridian of the affected organ.

1. Lung disorders (cough, asthma, panting): Lu 9, Lu 7, Lu 10, Lu 5, Lu 1.

2. Heart disorders (palpitation, insomnia, epilepsy): Ht 7, Ht 5, Ht 4.

3. Spleen disorders (diarrhea, abdominal pain and distention): Sp 4, Sp 6, Sp 15, Sp 16.

4. Kidney disorders (emission, incontinence of urine, impotence, edema): Ki 7, Ki 6, Ki 3, Ki 2.

5. Liver disorders (intercostal neuralgia, jaundice, hernia): Liv 3, Liv 2, Liv 1, Liv 13, Liv 14.

6. Pericardium disorders (angina, anxiety, epilepsy): Pc 8, Pc 7, Pc 6, Pc 2.

7. Stomach disorders (stomachache, vomiting, abdominal distention, indigestion, hiccough): St 36, St 37, St 44, St 34.

8. Urinary bladder disorders (incontinence of urine, oligurea): UB 28, UB 23, UB 26.

9. Gall bladder disorders (intercostal neuralgia, jaundice, gall stones): GB 24, GB 34, GB 40.

10. San Jiao disorders (intercostal neuralgia, chest fullness): TW 5, TW 6.

11. Large Intestine disorders (abdominal pain, incontinence of urine): L.I. 11, L.I. 7, L.I. 8, L.I.4.

12. Small Intestine disorders (lower abdominal pain, incontinence of urine): S.I. 1, S.I. 3, S.I. 8.

13. Conception Vessel disorder (leukorrhea): CV 3, CV 4, CV 6.

14. Governing Vessel Disorder (neck and back rigidity): GV 14, GV 3, GV 8, GV 4.

U. The Applied Prescribing Method of Yin/Yang Meridians

This prescription method chooses points either from both Yin and Yang meridians or from two Yang or two Yin meridians to enhance the treatment effect.

A. Yin meridian combined with Yang meridians for a balanced treatment:

1. Pc 6 and St 36:   vomiting and stomachache.

2. Sp 4 and St 36:   disorders of spleen and stomach

3. CV 12 and St 36: abdominal pain or distension and
                                   indigestion

4. Ht 6 and S.I. 3:   night sweats and restlessness

5. Ki 7 and L.I. 4 :   exogenous pathogenic heat without
                                   sweating

B. Yang meridian combined with a Yang meridian (two Yang meridians) to treat acute disorders frequently of a Yin nature:

1. L.I. 11 and St 36: various intestinal and stomach disorders
                                   and febrile diseases

2. L.I. 4 and TW 5:   most febrile diseases and disorders of
                                   the five sense organs

3. L.I. 4 and St 44:   toothache, painful and/or sore throat

4. TW 6 and GB 34: disorders of liver and gall bladder and
                                   intercostal neuralgia

C. Yin meridian combined with a Yin meridian (two Yin meridians)
   for chronic syndromes of a Yang nature.

1. SP 6 and Pc 6:   abdominal pain or distension and chest
                                   pain

2. Ht 7 and Sp 6:   insomnia

3. Ht 7 and Ki 3:   nightmare, insomnia and mental illness

V. The Applied Prescribing Method of Amounts of Qi and Blood

This method of prescription regards points according to the principle
of the relative amounts of Qi and Blood in the twelve meridians. The

amounts of Qi and Blood indicates the strength or weakness for adjusting the Qi and Blood in the twelve meridians. It is not related to the physiological or anatomical function of internal organs. The purpose of this method is to adjust tonification and dispersion in the treatment to keep the physiological function of internal organs in balance and to assist in recovery from disease. The following are the tables of the relative amounts of Qi and Blood in the twelve meridians.

Meridian	Amounts of Qi and Blood
L.I., Yangming-hand	more Qi and more Blood
St, Yangming - foot	
S.I., Taiyang - hand	
UB, Taiyang - foot	
Lu, Taiyin - hand	more Blood and less Qi
Sp, Taiyin - foot	
Pc, Jueyin - hand	
Liv, Jueyin - foot	
TW, Shaoyang - hand	
GB, Shaoyang - foot	more Qi and less Blood
Ht, Shaoyin - hand	
Ki, Shaoyin - foot	

Qi	Meridian	Blood	Location

YANG MERIDIANS

Qi	Meridian	Blood	Location
More	L.I.	More	
Less	S.I.	More	Hands
More	TW	Less	
More	St	More	
Less	UB	More	Feet
More	GB	Less	

YIN MERIDIANS

Qi	Meridian	Blood	Location
Less	Lu	More	
More	Ht	Less	Hands
Less	Pc	More	
Less	Sp	More	
More	Ki	Less	Feet
Less	Liv	More	

The principles underlying the balancing of Qi and Blood are applied to the prescribing method as follows:

1. In cases where the diagnosis is a syndrome of Qi Deficiency and/ or Qi Stagnation, the majority of points should be chosen from the meridians that have more Qi and less Blood, i.e.. TW, Ht, GB and Ki, along with some points from the St and L.I. meridians, if necessary. The tonification and/or dispersion of these points is based on the different kinds of syndromes.

2. In cases involving syndromes Blood Deficiency and/or Blood Stasis, the majority of points should be from the meridians that have more Blood and less Qi, i.e. Lu, Sp, Pc, S.I., Liv and UB,

plus some points from the St and L.I. meridians, if necessary. The tonification and/or dispersion of each point is again decided by the different kinds of syndromes diagnosed.

3. When treating patients diagnosed with Qi Stagnation and Blood Stasis the acupuncture prescription must consist of an equal number of points from each category. That is to say, if four points are selected from categories containing more Qi and less Blood, you must also needle four points from those categories which contains more Blood and less Qi, plus additional points from the St and L.I. meridians when necessary. As stated above, the tonification and/or dispersion of these points is decided by the nature of the syndrome.

W. The Applied Prescribing Method of Lower He Sea Points

This method employs the Lower He Sea Points of the three Yang meridians of the feet to treat disorders of the Six Fu organs (stomach, large intestine, small intestine, gall bladder, urinary bladder and sanjiao). For example, UB 54 (the Lower He Sea Point of the UB meridian) is chosen for treating urinary retention; St 37 (the Lower He Sea Points of the L.I. meridian) for colitis; St 39 (the Lower He Point of the S.I. meridian) for lower abdominal pain. The Lower He Sea Points can be used separately or in combination, for instance: GB 34 (the Lower He Sea Point of GB meridian) is chosen with CV 12, GB 24, GB 38, GB 36 for treating acute pain in the gall bladder due to gall stones or inflammatory conditions. In this case, CV 12 is chosen because the gall bladder is a Fu organ and CV 12 is an influential point for the Fu organs. GB 24 is a Mu Point of the gall bladder meridian (Mu Points are used for disorders of the Fu organs). GB 38 is a Fire point of the gall bladder (disperse GB 38 based on the mother-son relationship in excessive syndromes). GB 36 is the Xi point of the GB meridian (the Xi point is for acute disorders). The following are the Lower He Points and their indications:

1. St 36 (Yangming-foot): stomachache and acidity

2. St 37 (Yangming - foot): appendicitis and diarrhea

3. St 39 (Yangming-foot): lower abdominal pain and pain during urination

4. GB 34 (Shaoyang-foot): vomiting and pain in the gall bladder

5. UB 54 (Taiyang-foot): cystitis and retention of urine

6. UB 39 (Taiyang-foot): retention or urine and disorders of Sanjiao
    (stagnation of Qi in upper, middle and lower jiao)

X. The Applied Prescribing Method of Organ Phenomenon

This prescription method uses points according to the theories of chan-
nel-collateral and organ phenomenon. The prescribing principle is
the combination of Back Shu Points and their respectively related
Yuan-Luo Points. The following are the examples of how this method
is applied to treat each disorder of internal organs:

1. The liver stores blood and opens into the eye.

    a. Blurring of vision due to insufficiency of the Blood of the
        liver: UB 18 and Liv 3 (needle and moxibustion at both
        points).

    b. Red eye and flushed face due to flare-up of the Fire of
        liver: UB 18 and Liv 3 (dispersion technique or blood
        letting at both points).

2. The kidney stores essential substances and opens into the ear.
    The clinical sign of tinnitus due to insufficiency of kidney Yin:
    UB 23 and Ki 3 (needle and moxibustion at both points).

3. The lung determines skin and hair and opens into nose. The clini-
    cal signs of running nose and sore throat due to exogenous Wind/
    Cold: UB 13 and Lu 7 (needle and moxibustion at both points).

4. The heart determines blood and opens into tongue. The clinical
    sign of swelling and pain of the mouth and tongue: UB 15 and Ht
    7.

5. The spleen dominates muscle and opens into the mouth. The clini-
    cal signs of poor appetite, indigestion and light taste: UB 20 and
    Sp 4 (needle and moxibustion at both points).

Y. The Applied Prescribing Method Based on Syndromes

This method uses points according to the different kinds of syndromes in the process of disease. The following are the essential major prescriptions for various syndromes:

1. Fever: GV 14, L.I. 11, L.I. 4

2. Dizziness: GB 20, Liv 3, GV 20, Yintang

3. Insomnia: Ht 7, Sp 6, Ki 3

4. Nightmare: UB 15, Ht 7, Liv 3, St 36, Sp 6

5. Night Sweats: GV 14, S.I. 3, Ht 6

6. Cough: UB 14, UB 13, Lu 9

7. Excessive Sputum: St 40, UB 13, Lu 5

8. Shortness of breath: CV 6, St 36

9. Chest fullness or pain: Pc 6, Pc 5, TW 6

10. Intercostal Neuralgia: GB 34, TW 6

11. Sinusitis: L.I. 20, L.I. 4, L.I. 10

12. Nose bleeds: St 44, L.I. 4, Lu 11, GV 20

13. Tachycardia: Pc 6, Pc 5, Ht 6, St 32

14. Nausea or Vomiting: Pc 6, CV 12, Sp 4

15. Hemoptysis: St 34, GB 34, Pc 4

16. Stomachache: CV 12, St 34, Sp 4, Pc 6

17. Abdominal distention: Pc 6, St 36, St 43, L.I. 10

18. Abdominal Pain: CV 12, St 34, Sp 4, Pc 6

19. Ascites: CV 9, Ki 7

20. Diarrhea: St 25, Sp 9, St 36, L.I. 11

21. Constipation: TW 6, St 25, Ki 6

22. Urinary Retention: CV 3, Sp 9

23. Polyuria: CV 3, Ki 3, UB 23

24. Edema: St 28, Liv 13, St 36, Sp 9, Ki 7

25. Itching: L.I. 11, Sp 10, Sp 6

26. Muscle spasm: GB 34, L.I. 4, L.I. 11, GV 20

27. Weakness of body constitution: CV 4, CV 6, St 36

28. Bitter taste in the mouth: GB 38

29. Odorous in the mouth: Pc 7

30. Nocturnal enuresis: GB 23, UB 28, CV 3, Sp 6

Z. The Applied Prescribing Method Based on Differential Diagnosis

This method employs points according to the causative factors and the pathology of disease.

1. Invasion of the lung by exogenous pathogenic Wind-Cold or Wind-Heat.

Prescription:

   a. Wind-Cold (chills, nasal obstruction, watery nasal discharge, mucoid sputum, and a thin white tongue coating): UB 13 (Back Shu points), St 40 (Luo points), CV 17 (EIP, eight influential points), L.I. 20 (Lu —> L.I., exterior-interior relationship), Lu 7 (Luo point).

b. Wind-Heat (fever, purulent nasal discharge, purulent
    sputum, sore throat and a yellow tongue coating): Lu 10
    (Five Shu points), L.I. 5 (Five Shu points), St 40 (Luo
    points), CV 17 (EIP), L.I. 20 (Lu —> L.I.).

2. Stagnation of Liver Qi

    The patient has a syndrome of lower abdominal pain, breast dis-
    tention, chest fullness, irregular menstruation, and mental depres-
    sion.

Prescription: UB 18 (Shu-Mu points), Liv 14 (Shu-Mu points), Pc 6,
              Liv 3 (Pc —> Liv), TW 6, GB 31 (TW —> GB), CV 3,
              CV 6.

3. The heat retention of the Liver and Gall Bladder

    The patient has a syndrome of angry, unstable emotions and con
    vulsion.

Prescription: Liv 1 (Five Shu points), Liv 3, GB 31, GB 34 (Liv —>
              GB), UB 18 (Shu-Mu points), Liv 14 (Shu-Mu points).

4. Derangement of the mind

    The patient has a syndrome of mental confusion, depression and
    dullness. The purpose of treatment in this case is to clear the
    mind and harmonize the kidney and heart.

Prescription: UB 15 (Back Shu points), UB 23 (Back Shu points), Ki
              3, Ht 7 (Ht —> Ki), Sp 6 (the meeting place of Liv, Sp
              and Ki), Pc 6, Liv 3 (Pc —> Liv).

5. Deficiency and Cold of Spleen and Stomach

    The patient has a syndrome of indigestion, weakness, loose stool
    and vomiting of watery fluid.

Prescription: UB 20 (Back Shu point), UB 21 (Shu-Mu point),
              CV 12 (Shu-Mu points), Sp 4, St 25, St 36 (Sp <— St).

6. Deficiency of kidney Yang

The patient has a syndrome of chills, pallor, edema of the lower limbs, impotence, coldness of lower back and knee joints.

Prescription: UB 23 (Back Shu point), GV 4 and GV 20 (support and warm Kidney Yang), CV 4, CV 6, Sp 6, St 36 (Sp <— St).

7. Disharmony of Heart and Kidney

The patient has a syndrome of insomnia, depression, nightmare, mental confusion, unstable emotions and dreaming.

Prescription: UB 15, UB 23, Ht 6, Ht 7, Ki 3, Ki 6 (Ht —> Ki), Sp 6, Pc 6, CV 17.

8. Hyperactivity of Liver Fire

The patient has a syndrome of dizziness, red eyes, flushed face, headache and distending sensation of head.

Prescription: Sp 6, Ki 3, Ht 7 (Ki —> Ht), GV 20, GB 20, Liv 3.

PART THREE

ACUPUNCTURE

TECHNIQUES

Chapter I

The Basic Needle

Insertion Technique

CHAPTER I. THE BASIC NEEDLE INSERTION TECHNIQUE

Methods of Strengthening Your Fingers

To insert needles comfortably and efficiently, a practitioner must develop strength and dexterity of the fingers. This is called "finger force". With practice, the fingers acquire a familiarity in the handling of the needle that facilitates manipulation of the needle to regulate the qi.

A common practice method for beginning acupuncture students is to insert needles into different materials. The most common of these is a foam pad tied tightly with string or rubber bands to produce a surface that has resistance to pressure. Pin cushions such as those used for sewing are good for practice. Cotton batting rolled tightly into a ball or folded tissue paper tied tightly will also serve this purpose. See Figures 1 and 2.

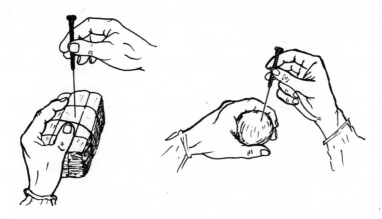

Figs. 1 & 2: Foam pad and pin cushion for strengthening fingers and
inserting needles

To practice needle insertion, hold the pad in one hand and the needle in the other. Your fingers must only touch the handle of the needle in accordance with Clean Needle Technique. Hold the needle firmly with the thumb and index finger. The third finger may be used at the handle if this feels natural to you. With a firm downward movement, press the needle through the surface of the pad to a depth of about 1/4". This penetration of the needle is the initial phase of needle insertion. See Figures 1 and 2.

In the human body, *needle penetration* of the first layer of skin is the *initial phase* of insertion. This is the level at which a sensation of pain may be felt, so this step should be done smoothly and quickly. The needle should be supported firmly in the skin and should not be flopping loosely to the side.

The *second phase* of insertion involves moving the needle downward to the property depth. The depth varies according to the location of the point. The needle can be rotated evenly as it is manipulated. The *final phase* of insertion is to *"obtain the qi"* or "Teh qi" and this includes a number of different movements described later in this section. These movements can all be practiced on a foam or cotton pad or pin cushion to develop "finger-force" and skill.

The Traditional Chinese Acupuncture Needle

The Chinese acupuncture needle is designed for smooth insertion and easy manipulation. It has five parts. See Figure 3.

1. Tip: The point of the needle. It is smooth and rounded and may be angled for a comfortable insertion. It is shaped like the tip of a pine cone. Unlike the sharp, cutting edges of needles used for injections, the tips of acupuncture needles are designed to slide through tissues without causing damage.

2. Body: The shaft of the needle which is uniform, solid and straight and is made of stainless steel wire of varied thicknesses.

3. Root: The juncture of the body of the needle and the handle.

4. Handle: Designed for gripping, the handle is made of wound wire. It may be of stainless steel, silver or copper and aluminum.

5. Tail: The circle and ring of the handle are designed to assist in gripping and manipulating the needle.

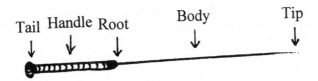

Fig. 3. The traditional Chinese acupuncture needle

Types of Needles

There are two basic types of Chinese needles, the filiform needle and the prismatic needle. The filiform needle is a slim and solid needle that is used in general clinical practice. The prismatic needle is a thicker needle with a sharp, three-edged tip used for bloodletting techniques. The plum blossom needle is a type of the prismatic needle that has either five or seven short points at the end of a handle. It is used to apply a technique called "cutaneous acupuncture" in which the surface of the body is treated for a superficial stimulation. See Figure 4.

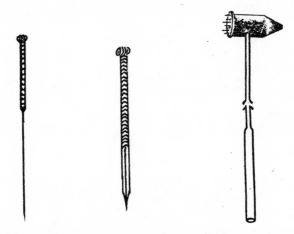

Fig. 4. The filiform needle, prismatic needle and plum needle

Filiform needles are made in a variety of lengths and gauges (thicknesses). The standard lengths are: 0.5 inch, 1.0 inch, 1.5 inch, 2.0 inch, 3.0 inch and 5.0 inch. The most commonly used lengths are 1.0 and 1.5 inch needles.

Needle gauges are designated as 26, 28, 30, 32, and 34. The 26 gauges needle is the thickest; the 34 gauge needle is the thinnest. The 30 gauge needle is the most often used in Chinese needle technique because it offers both stability for manual insertion and comfort of insertion for the patient.

The choice of needle length and gauge depends on the location of the point and the relative size of the patient. As a general guideline, shorter needles (0.5 inches) are used over thin musculature such as the head and face. Longer needles (1.5 and 2.0 inches) are used where the musculature is thicker, such as the hips and legs. One inch needles are good for use on the chest, abdomen and back where deeper insertions are prohibited to avoid puncturing of the internal organs.

The gauge needles used for Japanese acupuncture techniques are numbered by a different system. The following chart illustrates the comparisons between Chinese and Japanese needle gauges.

CHINESE	28 (gauge)	30	32	34
JAPANESE	10 (gauge)	8	6	4
Diameter	.34 (mm)	.30	.25	.22

The 28 gauge Chinese needle is thicker than the 30 gauge Chinese needle.

The 5 gauge Japanese needle is thicker than the 3 gauge Japanese needle.

The 30 gauge Chinese needle is equivalent in thickness to the 8 gauge Japanese needle.

CHINESE NEEDLE TECHNIQUES

The insertion of Chinese acupuncture needles requires skill to accomplish a comfortable and accurate insertion. An insertion technique will be selected based on several factors such as the thickness of the muscle at the puncture site, the presence of blood vessels, the surface tension of the skin, wrinkles or folds. There are three main types of insertion methods:

A. Rotation-Insertion Methods

These methods are the techniques used in the general practice of acupuncture. There are four basic techniques in this category, as well as several variation on these techniques. (See Figures 5, 6, 7 and 8). The four basic techniques are:

1. Two-finger Pressing Technique

2. Single-finger Pressing Technique

3. Spreading Skin Technique

4. Pinching Skin Technique

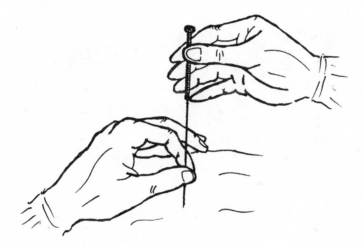

Fig. 5. Two-finger pressing technique

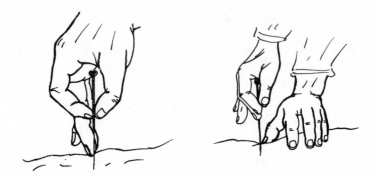

Fig. 6. Single-finger pressing technique

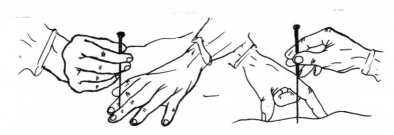

Fig. 7. Spreading skin technique

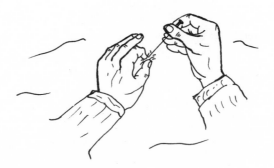

Fig. 8. Pinching skin technique

B. Stabbing Method

This technique is applied with the prismatic needle for the purpose of bloodletting. One hand holds a three-edged prismatic needle, or a lancet, while the other hand secures the skin at acupuncture point. The needle is quickly and firmly inserted to a depth of 0.6 to 1.0 cm and is immediately withdrawn. A small amount of bleeding at the puncture site is expected. This technique is used to reduce pathological Heat in the body and to circulate stagnant Blood.

C. Tube Insertion Method

With this technique, the needle is inserted into a thin tube that is slightly shorter in length than the needle.
The tube and needle is inserted into a thin tube that is slightly shorter in length than the needle. The tube and needle are placed over the point and held in place with one hand. The other hand is used to tap with the finger on the top of the needle causing it to enter the skin. The guide tube is then removed and the needle is inserted to the proper depth. This technique is most often used with very long needles as well as in the treatment of children and adults who are nervous about receiving acupuncture. See Figure 9.

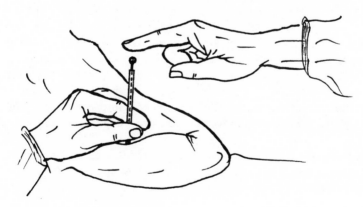

Fig. 9. Tube insertion method

Rotation-Insertion Technique

1. <u>Two-Finger Pressing Technique</u>
This technique is so named because both hands are used to perform the insertion. One hand holds a small piece of *sterile* cotton around the base of the needle while the other hand holds the needle at the handle. Together, both hands move the needle quickly downward to penetrate the skin. The cotton is then removed from the base and the needle is moved to the proper depth. See Figure 5.

The two-finger pressing technique offers the greatest control over longer needles (1.5 inches or more) since the body of the needle is supported by the fingers. Longer needles tend to bend under the pressure of insertion. It is very important that the fingers do not directly touch the body or the needle thereby compromising its sterility. The cotton used to hold the body of the needle must likewise be sterile cotton.

Longer needles are used where the musculature is thicker, such as the hips and legs. A special technique known as "threading", in which two consecutive points are connected with one needle through a horizontal insertion, also utilizes longer needles.

2. <u>Single-Finger Pressing Technique</u>
With this technique, one hand holds the needle at the handle and the other hand presses firmly on the skin next to the point. The pressing finger, usually the index finger, does not cover the point nor does it come into contact with any part of the needle. It serves to increase the surface tension of the skin at the point to aid insertion. The tip of the needle is placed lightly on the skin next to the pressing finger. A firm, downward movement allows the needle to penetrate the skin, after which the needle is moved to the correct depth. See Figure 6.

This technique is commonly used to insert needles one inch in length. This length needle does not require the extra support that the longer needles require.

Another application of this technique is the insertion of needles over blood vessels or where a pulse can be felt. The pressing finger covers the blood vessel pulling it gently to one side and the needle is inserted safely in front of the pressing finger. Similarly, the pressing finger covers the pulse thus protecting the underlying blood vessel from injury during insertion.

An advantage to the single-finger pressing technique is that the pressing finger feels comfortable to the patient and reduces the sensation of pain from insertion.

3. Spreading Skin Technique
This technique involves the use of the thumb and index fingers of one hand to stretch the skin taut on either side of the point to increase the surface tension. The other hand holds the needle and inserts it at the point with a firm, downward movement. See Figure 7.

There are two methods of holding the needle for this type of insertion. One method is to hold the needle a few millimeters from the tip with a piece of sterile cotton. The tip of the needle below the cotton is inserted into the point. With a second movement, the needle is held at the handle and moved to the correct depth. This is the easier method to use with the spreading skin technique. A second method involves holding the needle at the handle with the tip placed either above the skin or resting lightly on the skin. With a firm and quick downward movement, the needle is inserted with one hand while the other hand stretches the skin around the point. To do this technique with needles longer than one inch in length requires great skill.

Spreading skin technique is used to insert needles in an area of loose or wrinkled skin or folds in the skin such as at the elbow or on the abdomen or in the treatment of elderly patients.

4. Pinching Skin Technique
Here, the skin above the point is "pinched" or lifted with one hand making a tent. The other hand holds the needle with the tip of the needle placed lightly on the skin. The insertion is a firm movement into the pinched layer of skin. See Figure 8.

This technique is useful where the point is located over thin skin, such as on the face of Yintang, UB 2 (Zanzhu) or GB 14 (Yangbai). The insertion would be at an oblique angle since the skin is thin.

Specific Skills

ROTATION: With all of the rotation-insertion techniques, the needle may be rotated just after insertion to facilitate moving it to the proper depth. The tip of the needle is rounded for the purpose of gliding through skin and muscle tissue without causing injury. The movement of rotation with a small amplitude, slow frequency and even direction (equally rotated in both directions) eases the needle into position more comfortably than with simple, direct, downward pressure.

GRIP: The fingers must have a firm grip on the handle of the needle. The fingers must be able to press the needle into the point in a smooth and controlled manner. If their grip is weak and loose, the needle will not penetrate the skin and the patient will feel a painful sensation. If the needle is not firmly in place in the skin, it will fall over or fall out completely. To avoid this, *never let go of the handle of the needle* until the needle is supported firmly in the skin.

MOVEMENT: The movement of insertion should be definite, firm and quick. Hesitation on the part of the practitioner causes an insertion to be uncomfortable. Needle insertion is probably the most challenging skill for a beginner to master, so it is important to be prepared and to feel confident before attempting the insertion.

Angles of Insertion

There are three angles at which the needle may be inserted into the point (See Figure 10):

1. Perpendicular: the needle forms a 90 degree angle with the skin.
2. Oblique: the needle forms a 45 degree angle with the skin.
3. Transverse: the needle forms a 15 to 25 degree angle with the skin.

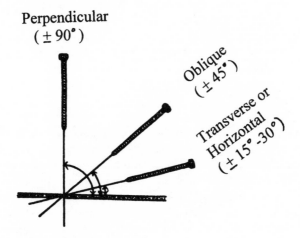

Fig. 10. The angles of insertion

The angle of insertion that is most commonly used over muscle tissue is the perpendicular insertion. The oblique angle is used where the musculature is thin or where the point lies above the organs or blood vessels. The transverse insertion is used where the skin is very thin, such as over bone on the head, the face and the chest.

Most texts describe the angle of insertion that is indicated for each point. Different angles of insertion can be applied at the same point to achieve different therapeutic effects. For example, SI 11 (Tianzong) may be needled perpendicularly to address pain in the scapula. Or, the needle may be directed obliquely toward the neck to address pain in that area; pain in the shoulder can be treated with SI 11 by directing the needle toward the shoulder area. This illustrates the concept of needling in the direction of pain.

Depth of Insertion

The depth of insertion depends on the location of the point, the condition of the patient and the quality of needle sensation that the patient experiences. Each point has a recommended depth of insertion that corresponds to the thickness of the muscle or tissue over which the point is located. Beyond this consideration, there are other factors to consider. In a patient who is very weak, the qi may be very

deep within the body and a deeper insertion would be required to
regulate the qi. Similarly, in a patient with strong qi, a relatively shallow insertion may produce a strong qi sensation. Once the qi sensation has been obtained, it is not usually necessary to move the needle
to a deeper level.

Qi Sensation

After inserting the needle to the proper depth, the needle will be in
contact with the qi. The patient will feel a distinct sensation often
described as soreness, numbness, heaviness or distention around the
point. This is known as "qi sensation". It is a distinctly different feeling from the sensation of pain. The acupuncturist can often sense
when the qi has been obtained. Holding firmly onto the handle of the
needle and concentrating on the acupuncture point, the acupuncturist
can sense when the qi has been stimulated by the needle. There is a
tightening or a tenseness around the needle, which is known as "the
arrival of qi," or "Teh qi".

Some acupuncture points are characteristically subtle in qi sensation
and others are strong. The qi sensation also varies from patient to
patient. If there is no needle sensation during the treatment of a patient with a weak constitution or a chronic illness, it is possible that
therapeutic results will not be attained.

If no qi sensation is felt, the practitioner should check the point location to be sure that it is accurate. The needle can be re-angled without
removing it completely. Withdraw the needle to just below the skin
and redirect it at a different angle. If still no qi sensation is felt, the
practitioner would want to "induce the arrival of qi".

There are a number of techniques that can be used to induce the arrival of qi (see Figures 11, 12, 13, and 14):

1. Rotation: the needle is rotated quickly back and forth.

2. Scraping: the handle of the needle is scraped with the nail from
               the root to the tail using the thumb or index finger at
               the top of the handle to stabilize the needle.

3. Vibrating: the needle is raised and lowered with small amplitude and rapid speed to cause the needle to vibrate, tremble or shake.

4. Flicking: the tail of the needle is "flicked" with the nail of the index or middle finger.

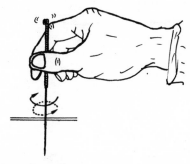

Fig. 11. The rotation of needle

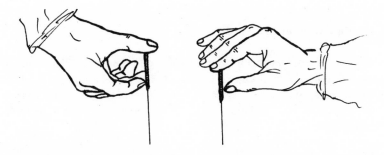

Fig. 12. Scraping needle

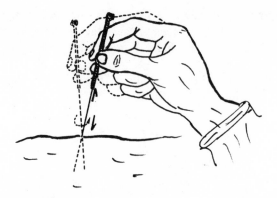

Fig. 13. Vibrating needle

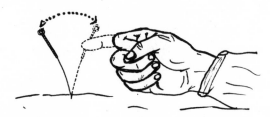

Fig. 14. Flicking needle

Manipulation of the Needle

After the needle has been inserted, moved to the correct depth and qi
sensation has been obtained, the needle can then be manipulated for
therapeutic effects. The effects of needle manipulation are that of
"tonification" and "dispersion". There are three categories of manipulation methods:

1. Tonification method:

   a. Effect: to correct the deficiency of vital function and
           strengthen body resistance.

   b. Indications: deficient conditions, chronic conditions, non-
           febrile conditions.

2. Dispersion method:

    a. Effect: to eliminate the excess of pathogenic factor.

    b. Indications: excess conditions; acute conditions with fever and distinct symptoms.

3. Even method:

    a. Effect: to treat diseases which involve both deficiency and excess

    b. Indications: diseases that are both "hot" and "cold", both "deficient" and "excess".

In addition to needle technique being reinforcing, reducing or even in therapeutic effect, some points have specific properties with regards to tonification and dispersion. For example, needling points St 36, CV 4, UB 23 will have a *reinforcing* effect in promoting functional activity. Needling points UB 54 and Pc 3 in order to reduce fever and expel an excess pathogenic factor will have a *reducing* or dispersing effect.

Needle Stimulation

There are three degrees of needle stimulation: strong, moderate and mild stimulation.

1. Strong Stimulation:

    a. Technique: manipulation of the needle is strong and energetic.

    b. Sensation: the patient feels a strong qi sensation locally and in distal areas.

    c. Application: acute, painful disorders; patients with a strong constitution and no fear of needles. This stimulation is usually used at points on the four limbs.

2. Moderate Stimulation:

   a. Technique: manipulation of the needle is steady, regular
                    and moderate.

   b. Sensation: the patient feels a mild sensation around the
                    needle locally and sometimes in distal areas as
                    well.

   c. Application: for general use.

3. Mild or Weak Stimulation:

   a. Technique: manipulation of the needle is slow and gentle
                    and movements are shallow.

   b. Sensation: the patient feels a slight sensation around the
                    needle.

   c. Application: weakened conditions; needle-shy or nervous
                   patients. This stimulation is appropriate for use
                   over major internal organs.

Precautions

The following is a list of general precautions to consider in the use of
acupuncture:

1. Delay treatment or use only a few needles if the patient is hungry
    or has over-eaten, and if the patient is intoxicated, exhausted or
    in a very weakened condition.

2. The fontanel of infants should not be needled.

3. Do not needle points located on the abdomen and lumbo-sacral
    region of a pregnant woman in the first trimester. After three
    months, avoid the upper abdomen as well. Points causing strong
    sensation (such as LI 4, SP 6, UB 60, UB 67, CV 3, CV 4 and CV
    6) are forbidden to needle on the pregnant patient.

4. Specific points are forbidden to needle because of their location

near vital organs or large blood vessels. It is important to know the needling cautions or contraindications according to the literature.

5. Check your needle for hooks or burrs on the tip of the needle and check that the body of the needle is straight and not bent.

6. It is recommended that needles used for electro-acupuncture be used only once due to the weakening effect of electricity on metals.

7. Acupuncture for children requires the use of much shallower depths, usually 0.2-0.3 cun. It is important that children keep still during treatment to aid insertion and manipulation of the needles and to avoid bending the needles during treatment.

Preparation for Acupuncture Treatment

<u>Wash</u> your hands with soap under warm running water for a minimum of 10 seconds before beginning to work with the patient.

<u>Prepare</u> your equipment for treatment. In the treatment room, you will need to have on a treatment cart or on an instrument tray:

> Needle dish; Cotton jar for clean cotton; Needles and cotton in a sterile package for each patient; Alcohol; Sterile forceps; Moxa (loose moxa, moxa pole, etc.); Lighter; Bowl for moxa ash; and Biohazard container.

Other equipment may be required for different techniques.

<u>Inform</u> your patient about the procedure you will be doing and ask if s/he is comfortable and relaxed and if s/he has any questions.

<u>Position</u> the patient for treatment. The patient should always be relaxed and comfortable for the duration of the treatment (30-45 minutes). The position of the patient is determined by which area of the body is to be needled according to the points selected.

1. Sitting on a chair: for treating the head, neck, shoulders and extremities.

2. Lying in supine position: for treating the face, head, chest, abdomen and extremities.

3. Lying in prone position: for treating the back and the back of the leg.

4. Lying in lateral recumbent position: for treating the hip joint, and back.

CLINICAL COMPLICATIONS IN THE PRACTICE OF ACUPUNCTURE

Stuck Needle

One of the more common clinical experiences in the practice of acupuncture is that of a needle being difficult to remove, or a "stuck needle". Muscle fibers around the needle tighten up and hold the needle in place. There are a number of reasons why this could happen:

1. Excessive force of insertion

2. Uneven manipulation

3. Muscle spasm (involuntary)

4. Muscle cramp which may occur if the patient is in pain or if the needle has been retained for too long in a muscle

5. Muscle contraction caused by the patient moving suddenly which may occur if the patient is tense or extremely nervous.

Management

It is not difficult to remove a stuck needle and there are several methods to try. Remain calm and keep the patient relaxed.

1. Wait a few minutes for the muscle to relax and the needle may loosen.

2. Lightly press into the muscle around the needle near the point.

3. Apply a warm moistened cloth.

4. Insert another needle 1-2 inches away: this "scatters the accumulation of qi and blood".

5. Rotate needle in the opposite direction with small amplitude.

6. For a needle that has bent beneath the skin:

    a. lightly shake the needle from side to side.

    b. look at the direction of the handle to determine the direction of bend and pull in the same direction.

    c. never force the needle.

To prevent a needle from becoming stuck during treatment, perform careful insertions and manipulations. Explain to the patient to remain still while the needles are in place. Finally, inspect needles regularly for burrs or hooks at the tip or along the body.

Broken Needle

Acupuncture needles must be of good quality to avoid breakage during treatment. If there are imperfections in the body of the needle such as cracks, erosions, hooks or burrs or the needle is loose at the root (the juncture of the body and the handle), there is the risk of it breaking while in place. Other causes of a broken needle are: a strong muscle spasm; manipulation of the needle that is too forceful; using excessive force while withdrawing a needle; manipulating a stuck needle too forcefully; or the patient moving suddenly.

Management

1. Remain calm.

2. Keep patient still.

3. Extract with forceps, tweezers or hemostat if the needle protrudes above the skin.

4. If needle is at the level of the skin: press with the thumb and index finger against the skin surrounding the needle and grasp with forceps, tweezers or hemostat.

5. If the needle is broken deep in the tissue: remove surgically.

To avoid having a broken needle, inspect needles for irregularities. Explain to the patient to be still during treatment and stay in the room with patients who are very nervous or in great pain. *Never insert a needle up to the root of the handle.* It is recommended that 0.3 – 0.5 inch of the body of the needle be above the skin.

Fainting

Fainting during treatment can happen as the result of excessive nervousness, fatigue, weakness, hunger or too strong and excessive manipulation of the needle.

This kind of loss of consciousness is called "psychogenic shock" and is a nervous system reaction. (It is not neurogenic shock which is a failure of the nervous system to control the diameter of blood vessels as seen with spinal cord injury.) In fainting, a sudden dilation of the blood vessels take place and the proper blood flow to the brain is momentarily interrupted. This is a temporary condition and is considered a self-correcting form of shock. It is important to remember that the patient has not suffered an injury and will likely recover on his or her own in a few minutes.

The symptoms of fainting are:

dizziness	vertigo
pallor	palpitations
nausea	oppressive feeling in chest

If severe, there may be:

cold extremities	cold sweating
weak pulse	loss of cosnciousness
cyanosis	hypotension
incontinence	shock

Management

1   Stop needling when symptoms first appear.

2   Remove needles.

3. Have the patient lay down with the head slightly lower than the feet since this helps blood circulation to the brain.

4. Loosen tight clothing.

5. Offer a warm beverage.

6. Allow the patient to recover on his/her own unless signs of distress develop such as difficulty breathing.

7. Remain with the patient until s/he has recovered (look for facial color, a stronger pulse, relaxed breathing, mentally alert and oriented, etc.)

8. If the patient has fainted:

    a. firmly press GV 26 with fingernail, or needle GV 26 and Pc 6.

    b. firmly press, moxa or needle ST 36 if needling has been done in the upper half of the body, and LI 4 if in the lower half.

    c. needle or press hard with the fingernail at GV 26, LI 4 or Ki 1; or

    d. use smelling salts to revive and allow the patient to rest.

To prevent the likelihood of a patient fainting, treat patients lying down if they are weak, tired, fasting or in a nervous state. Needle manipulation on these patients should be gentle. Observe facial expression and color for any unusual changes. Hungry patients should eat before treatment. Discuss procedures with nervous patients before proceeding. The treatment room should have proper ventilation.

If a patient is treated in a sitting position, give him or her support with cushions or blankets.

Generally, the patient will respond to these measures, but if the symptoms are still unrelieved, call for emergency medical assistance.

Injury to Organs

Lung–

Pneumothorax is a condition that results when air enters the thoracic cavity and is trapped in the pleural space. Air can enter through an external wound opening or may escape internally from a punctured lung. In pneumothorax, the injured lung collapses. Air accumulates on the injured side and can force the heart against the uninjured lung.

Pneumothorax can occur if an acupuncture needle is inserted too deeply or in an incorrect direction in the region of the lungs, specifically the supraclavicular fossa, the thorax and the upper back. If an acupuncture needle punctures the pleura, air can enter the pleural sac; if it punctures the lung, air escapes internally into the thoracic cavity. The flow of air through a needle track may be slow and symptoms may not appear for several hours.

In treating coughs or asthma, there is the risk of the needles moving during treatment, when the patient's chest moves (from coughing or labored breathing) and special care must be taken not to needle too deeply. In slender patients, the apex of the lung may be as little as 2 cm from the surface of the body. Caution is advised in treating the lung region in patients with a history of spontaneous pneumothorax in which the lung can, to some degree, collapse without any apparent injury.

Symptoms

The symptoms of a pneumothorax are:

    pain or a sensation of fullness in the chest
    cyanosis
    sweating
    hypotension

coma and other symptoms associated with shock
coughing up of bright red frothy blood indicates a punc-
    tured lung
difficult breathing
pallor

Management

1. Withdraw the needle immediately: the worst damage is
    tearing of tissue done by breathing or coughing while the
    needle is in place.

2. Let the patient rest calmly.

3. Take the patient to the hospital or call for emergency
    medical assistance.

4. In some cases the patient will show no signs of trouble
    until hours later when chest pain and breathing difficulties
    may appear.

Puncturing the lung is entirely avoidable if the acupuncturist adheres
strictly to the recommendations for proper depth and angle of insertion. Slanted or transverse insertions are recommended for areas over
the lung.

Caution is advised in needling specific points such as: CV 22, GB
21, UB 12, UB 13, UB 14, UB 15, Liv 14.

Brain And Spinal Cord–

Needling too deeply or at the wrong angle at points between and be-
side the upper cervical vertebrae involves the risk that the medulla
oblongata may be punctured. Improper needling of points between
the thoracic vertebrae could present damage to the spinal cord.

Symptoms

The symptoms of a puncture to the medulla oblongata are:

post-treatment symptoms of headache, nausea, vomiting or
    disorientation may be the first indications
convulsions
severe bleeding
paralysis
coma

The symptoms of a puncture to the spinal cord are:

an electric, flash pain that can be felt in the extremities

Management

Needling must be stopped immediately to avoid continued pain after
treatment. If symptoms are prolonged and severe, the patient should
see a physician.

Again, proper use of needle angle and depth of insertion can prevent
this type of injury.

Caution is advised in needling specific points as: CV15; CV16; GB
20.

Heart, Liver, Spleen and Kidney–

The treatment of points in the region of the abdomen requires the
knowledge of the location of the internal organs. Needling too deeply
could puncture the heart, liver, spleen or kidney.

Symptoms

If injury to the spleen or liver:

pain felt locally and often extending toward the back
abdominal rigidity

If injury to the kidney:

pain around the waist
blood in the urine

If serious bleeding occurs, there will be a drop in the blood pressure and shock may follow.

Management

1. If the damage is minor, it will usually heal itself with rest.

2. If there is bleeding, the patient must be monitored (observed) for blood pressure, pulse, respiration, temperature, etc.; a cold compress may be applied to stop bleeding. If serious, hospitalize.

These kinds of injuries are preventable if the practitioner knows the anatomical locations of the organs and the points. Perform a physical exam of the patient before needling to determine if there are enlargements of the organs. A medical evaluation should identify any internal abnormalities.

Nerve Trunk–

Damage to a nerve trunk can occur if a needle mistakenly punctures a nerve bundle or nerve plexus.

Symptoms

Flash pain (a strong, distinct, jolting type pain sensation) to the extremities.

If a nerve trunk is directly stimulated by a needle, a flash pain extending to the extremities will be felt. If stimulation is continued, damage to the nerve tissue could result in peripheral neuritis with symptoms of continued pain and numbness, or functional impairment along the pathway of the nerve.

Management

1. In superficial cases: light massage.

2. In serious cases: Vitamin B complex injections by a physician.

This type of injury is preventable if needle technique is done with care. Be aware of the difference between a pain sensation and a qi sensation.

Local Hematoma–

A hematoma results when capillaries are punctured and a small amount of bleeding occurs. Blood accumulates in a small area producing a lump beneath the skin or causes bruising or discoloration of the skin.

Symptoms

> bleeding at the point
> ache or soreness at the site
> a lump
> a bruise

Management

1. Normally a hematoma will resolve itself within a few days.

2. If there is discomfort, apply a cold compress followed by a hot compress or indirect moxa to stop the bleeding and disperse the accumulation of blood.

To prevent bruising, check the needle tip for hooks or burrs; examine the skin for local capillaries and blood vessels before needling; and be careful needling elderly patients whose blood vessel walls have less elasticity.

Accidents do not happen very often but care must be taken to prevent them. Have emergency telephone numbers of a physician and emergency medical assistance on hand. If a clinical complication does arise, remain calm yourself and try to calm your patient. Make a sincere effort to remedy the situation and assure the patient's well-being. And keep in close contact with the patient personally to know what is being done and to offer your support.

BLOODLETTING

"When the flow of qi and blood is impeded and the channels are obstructed, bleeding should be effected by needling." — from *Simple Questions*

Bloodletting is a "stabbing" technique that causes bleeding at acupuncture points or superficial blood vessels so as to reduce heat, activate the blood and reduce swelling. The needle used in bloodletting is called a "prismatic needle", is a "pyramid needle", or a "three-edge needle" and has a triangular shape with sharp edges. (See Figure 4) Also used are thick filiform needles. Lancets are sterilized disposable bleeding needles that have a plastic handle for gripping.

Technique

The use of protective gloves is important for the safe practice of this technique.

1.   Apply pressure to the area to increase circulation. If you are bleeding the Jing-Well points (see page 165), for example, hold the finger firmly and press from the base to the end of the finger until it reddens slightly.

2   Clean the area to be needled with alcohol.

3.   Insert the needle with a swift downward movement and withdraw the needle with equal speed. The depth of insertion is 0.1 inch deep. The size of the puncture should be small.

4.   Allow a few drops of blood to escape. Have sterile cotton ready to absorb the blood. A small amount of blood is desired. If blood flow is minimal, press gently 1-2 inches away from the puncture to encourage local circulation.

5.   Press the point with sterile cotton to stop the bleeding.

6.   Clean the area with alcohol.

If you are using a prismatic needle, you may wrap the base of the needle with a small piece of cotton at the desired depth of insertion.

Hold the needle at the base with your fingers over the cotton.

It is important to thoroughly clean the area of the puncture with alcohol both before and after bloodletting to avoid infection.

Indications

tonsillitis	sore throat
allergic dermatitis	heatstroke
febrile diseases	rhinitis
eczema	numbness of the fingers or toes
hematoma	phlebitis
coma	neurodermatitis
mental disorders	abscesses
sprain	acute conjunctivitis or keratitis
headache	lymphangitis
erysipelas	hemorrhoids

Precautions

1. Patients with hemorrhagic diseases or vascular tumors should not have bloodletting done.

2. Use extreme caution in applying bloodletting in the treatment of patients who are weak, anemic, hyposensitive and in the treatment of pregnant or post-partum women.

Application

The following are examples of some uses of the prismatic needle in treatment.

Acute Tonsillitis
Prick Lu 11 to disperse wind and heat along the lung channel; prick Li 1 if treatment is directed toward dispersing heat.

Headache
For "overheating headache" that presents with signs of red face and a strong pulse due to fire in the upper part of the body, prick Pc 9, Li 1, If severe, prick GV 20.

If the headache starts at the same time every day, bleed the Jing-Well points on the fingers or toes according to which meridian is associated.

High Blood Pressure (Affecting Brain)
Prick GV 20 and Pc 9.

Yang Madness (mental disorder)
Prick the Jing-Well points and the Luo points (see pages 165, 177). The Jing points are commonly used for bloodletting because they regulate the qi of the 12 primary channels.

Bronchitis
For treatment of dry cough, prick Lu 11.

Heat Exhaustion or Sunstroke
Prick the Jing-Well points and Pc 3 and UB 54 to drain heat.

Chronic Lack of Appetite in Children
Prick the middle creases of the four fingers and press out the liquid that is there (a glue or gum-like substance); prick Ht 8 in the same manner.

Influenza
For high temperature, prick Li 4, Lu 11 and Pc 9.

Epistaxis
Bleed Lu 11 and GV 23.

Again, these procedures are only part of a treatment plan and not treatments that stand alone (see page 177, apply Luo points in bloodletting).

Chapter II

The Basic Methods for

Tonification and Dispersion

CHAPTER II. THE BASIC METHODS FOR TONIFICATION AND DISPERSION

Acupuncturists from ancient times through today have recognized that the techniques of tonification and dispersion are the most important part of acupuncture technique. The *Nei Jing (Esoteric Book)* dating from 1,200-4,000 B.C., the first written record of Chinese Medicine, indicated that "diseases have deficient and excessive syndromes and, therefore, tonification and dispersion are required in acupuncture treatment. The needle, after insertion but without manipulation, is like a tree after planting in the earth without water or fertilizer. Proper manipulation of the needle produces remarkable results, but these results are dependent upon the skillful technique of the manipulation".

When the needle has been inserted at the point, the QI sensation must be obtained before beginning to operate the techniques for tonification and dispersion. This is known as "Teh Qi", which is a needle sensation that occurs when the Qi connects to the needle. It is like the feeling of "a fish taking a hook" when one is fishing. The patient will feel a needle sensation of soreness, numbness, cold, heat or distension. By lightly moving the needle up and down or scratching the handle of the needle after insertion, the acupuncturist can obtain the Qi sensation or, "Teh Qi". If the patient is suffering from a prolonged illness and weakness due to Qi deficiency, the Qi will be slow to arrive after needling at the point. The acupuncturist should wait for the arrival of the Qi before proceeding with the proper technique for tonification and dispersion to enhance the therapeutic effect.

A. Twist Method

The principle of this method is to rotate the needle in the direction of clockwise or counterclockwise based on the pathway of meridians to enhance or decline the Qi circulation in the meridians for the function of tonification and dispersion.

The fourteen meridians are divided into two groups based on the direction of the meridians for practice of this method. In Group I, the pathway of the meridians is from down to up; in Group II, the direction is from up to down.

Group I	3 Yang (hands)	L.I.	S.I.	T.W.	up
	3 Yin (feet)	Sp	Ki	Liv	
	CV, GV				down

| Group II | 3 Yin (hands) | Lu | Ht | Pc | up |
| | 3 Yang (feet) | St | UB | GB | down |

1. Tonification of the points in Group I

    Rotate the needle in a counterclockwise direction. Do this
    by twisting the needle back and forth between the thumb
    and index finger and rolling the needle back up toward the
    tip of the thumb with the index finger. The following
    figure shows the direction of movement of the thumb and
    index finger for tonification using the twist method for

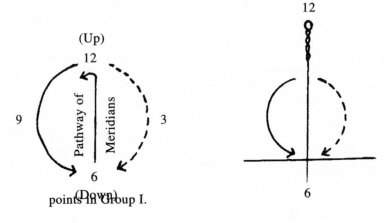

    points in Group I.

    Solid arrow: Thumb (forceful rotation)
    Broken arrow: Index finger (gentle rotation)

2. Dispersion of the points inGroup I

    Rotate the needle in a clockwise direction. Twist the
    needle back and forth between the thumb and the index
    finger (rolling the needle back up toward the tip of the
    index finger with the thumb). The following diagram
    shows the direction of movement of the thumb and index

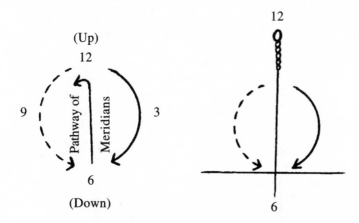

finger for dispersion using the twist method in Group I.
Solid arrow: Index finger (forceful rotation)
Broken arrow: Thumb (gentle rotation)

3.   Tonification of the points in Group II

Rotate the needle in a clockwise direction (twist the needle
back and forth between the thumb and index finger while
rolling the needle back up toward the tip of the index
finger with the thumb). The following diagram shows the
direction of movement of your thumb and index finger for

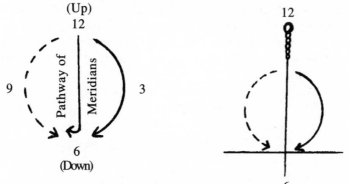

tonification with the twist method in Group II.

Solid arrow: Index finger (forceful rotation)

Broken arrow: Thumb (gentle rotation)

4. Dispersion of the points in Group II

Rotate the needle in a counterclockwise direction (twist the
needle back and forth between the thumb and index finger;
roll the needle back up toward the tip of the thumb with
index finger). The following diagram shows the direction
of movement of the thumb and index fingers for dispersion

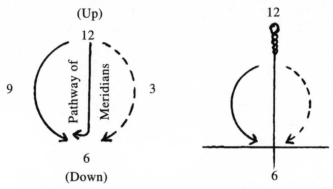

using the twist method in Group II.
Solid arrow: Thumb (forceful rotation)
Broken arrow: Index finger (gentle rotation)

B. Lift and Thrust Method

The principle of this method is to plant the Wei Qi (Defensive Qi)
from the exterior to the interior part of the body for tonification and
to take out the pathogenic Qi from the interior to the exterior part of
the body for dispersion by gently, slowly, heavily or quickly moving
the needle up or down.

1. Tonification

   Forcefully and quickly thrust the needle into the point and
   gently and slowly lift the needle up.

   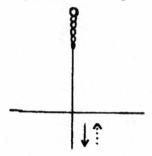

   Solid arrow: Forceful and quick movement
   Broken arrow: Gentle and slow movement

2. Dispersion

   Gently and slowly thrust the needle into the point and
   forcefully and quickly exit the needle up.

   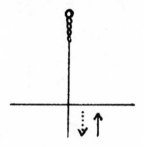

   Solid arrow: Forceful and quick movement
   Broken arrow: Gentle and slow movement

C. The Respiratory Method

The principle of this method involves insertion and manipulation of the needle during exhalation or inhalation for tonification
and dispersion. This method is suitable for the points located on
the trunk or thick muscle areas.

1. Tonification

    a. Massage around the points before inserting needle.

    b. The needle is inserted during exhalation (Fig C-1) and held while waiting for the Qi to arrive or manipulate to hasten its arrival.

    c. Keep the needle still during inhalation (Fig C-2).

    d. When the Qi has arrived, the needle should be twisted slightly (see twist method) during exhalation (C-3).

    e. Repeat steps c and d for several periods of time such as every ten minutes.

    f. Withdraw the needle during inhalation (Fig C-4) and press the needle hole gently with a cotton ball.

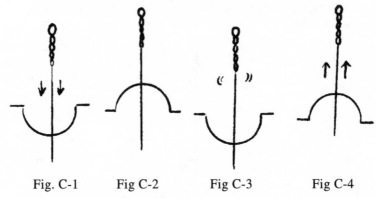

Fig. C-1   Fig C-2   Fig C-3   Fig C-4

2. Dispersion

    a. Massage around the point before inserting needle

    b. The needle is inserted during inhalation (Fig C-5) and held while waiting for the Qi to arrive or it is manipulated to hasten its arrival.

    c.   Keep the needle still during exhalation (Fig C-6)

    d.   After the Qi arrived the needle should be twisted slightly (see twist method) during inhalation (Fig C-7)

    e.   Repeat steps c and d for several periods of the time, such as every ten minutes.

    f.   Withdraw the needle during exhalation (Fig C-8) and keep the needle hole open.

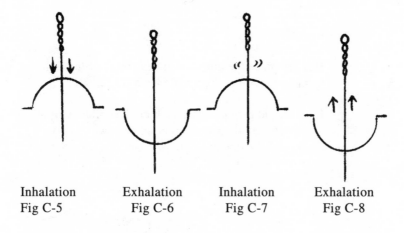

Inhalation	Exhalation	Inhalation	Exhalation
Fig C-5	Fig C-6	Fig C-7	Fig C-8

D. Scratch Method

The principle of this method is the same as that in the lift and thrust method. This method is good to hasten the arrival of Qi.

1.   Tonification

    a.   Apply a slight force to the top of the needle head with the thumb of the left hand; hold the needle body with the backs of the index fingers of both hands (Fig D-1).

    b.   Repeatedly scratch on the coiled wire of needle handle in the direction of up to down with the nail of thumb of right hand (Fig D-1).

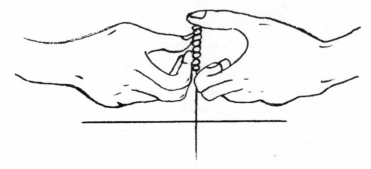

Fig D-1

2. Dispersion

    a. Heavily place the thumb or index finger of the right
        hand on the top of the needle head (Fig D-2).

    b. Heavily and repeatedly scratch on the coiled wire of
        the needle handle in the direction of down to up with
        the nail of the thumb or index finger of the right hand
        (Fig. D-2 and D-3).

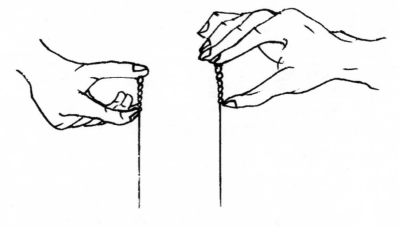

Fig D-2   Fig. D-3

E. Slow and Quick Method

The principle of this method is to support of preserve the antipathogenic Qi or eliminate the pathogenic Qi by inserting or withdrawing the needle slowly or quickly

1. Tonification

    a.   Insert the needle slowly to a certain depth.

    b.   Manipulate the needle based on the twist or lift and thrust method for tonification.

    c.   Withdraw the needle quickly whenever the needle has to be taken out, then press the needle hole gently with a cotton ball.

2. Dispersion

    a.   Insert the needle quickly to a certain depth.

    b.   Manipulate the needle based on the twist or lift and thrust method for dispersion.

    c.   Withdraw the needle slowly whenever the needle has to be taken out, then keep the needle hole open.

Chapter III

The Comprehensive Methods for

Tonification and Dispersion

CHAPTER III THE COMPREHENSIVE METHODS FOR TONIFICATION AND DISPERSION

The application of the comprehensive methods for tonification and dispersion is based on various basic methods, and their principles have evolved from the principles of the basic methods. The techniques that are described in this chapter emphasize the use of these methods for treatment of the following conditions:

1. The syndromes of cold first, then heat (the syndromes of deficiency associated with excess), for example, asthma, the common cold, cough, diarrhea, abdominal pain, insomnia and Bi-syndrome.

2. The syndromes of heat first, then cold (the syndromes of excess associated with deficiency), for example, asthma, the common cold, cough, diarrhea, abdominal pain, insomnia and Bi-syndrome.

3. Intense painful syndromes.

4. The lack of clarity in the deficient and excessive syndromes.

5. The various persistent disorders.

Waiting for and hastening the arrival of the Qi for those methods is required when applying the comprehensive method for tonification and dispersion in treating the above syndromes.

A. Yang Concealed Yin Method

1. Principle:

    The manipulation of tonification and dispersion at the same time is indicated for treatment of the condition of cold first and heat later or for treating the syndromes of deficiency associated with excess.

2. Contains:

    a. Slow and quick method
    b. Lift and thrust method

3. Indications:

Disorders with a syndrome of cold first with heat later (deficiency associated with excess), for example, asthma, common cold, cough, diarrhea, abdominal pain, insomnia and Bi-syndrome.

4. Method:

    a. Insert the needle to O.5 cun (shallow part of inserting depth) and wait for the arrival of Qi

    b. Heavily and quickly move the needle down to 1.0 cun (the shallow part) and gently and slowly move the needle up to 0.5 cun for a total of nine times for tonification (Fig. A-1)

    c Move the needle down to 1.0 cun.

    d. Gently and slowly move the needle down to 1.5 - 2 cun (the deepest level of insertion depth) and heavily and quickly move the needle up to 1.0 cun for a total of six times for dispersion (Fig A-1).

    e. Move the needle up to 0.5 cun.

    f. Repeat steps b, c, d, and e if necessary.

The different depths of 0.5 cun, 1.0 cun or 1.5 cun indicate the depth of needle insertion in the muscle. Thus, you have to divide the thickness of the muscle into two parts (shallow and deep), depending on the point location.

The needle is manipulated in the shallow part first and the deep part later. If, for example, the acupuncture point is located on a muscle that is 3 cun thick, the shallow part is between 0.5 - 1.5 cun, and the deep part is between 1.5 - 3 cun.

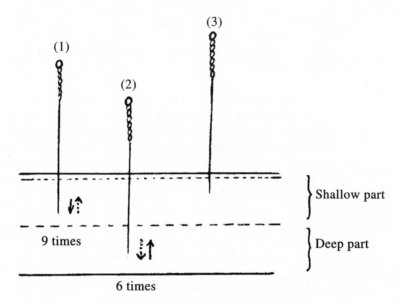

Fig. A-1 Yang concealed Yin method

B. Yin Concealed Yang Method

1. Principle:

    The manipulation of dispersion and tonification at the
    same time is for treating the condition of heat first and
    cold later or for treating the syndromes of excess associ-
    ated with deficiency.

2. Contains:

    a. Slow and quick method
    b. Lift and thrust method.

3. Indications:

    Disorders with the heat syndrome first and the cold
    syndrome later (excess associated with deficiency), for
    example, asthma, common cold, cough, diarrhea, abdomi-
    nal pain, insomnia and Bi-syndrome.

4. Method:

   a. Insert the needle to a depth of 1.0 cun and wait for the
       Qi to arrive.

   b. Gently and slowly move the needle down to 1.5 - 2
       cun (the deepest part of needle insertion) and heavily
       and quickly move the needle up to 1 cun for a total of
       six times for dispersion (Fig B-1)

   c. Move the needle up to 0.5 cun (the shallow part of
       needle insertion).

   d. Heavily and quickly move the needle down to 1 cun
       and gently and slowly move the needle up to 0.5 cun
       for a total of nine times for tonification (Fig B-1)

   e. Move the needle down to 1 cun.

   f. Repeat steps b, c, d and e if necessary.

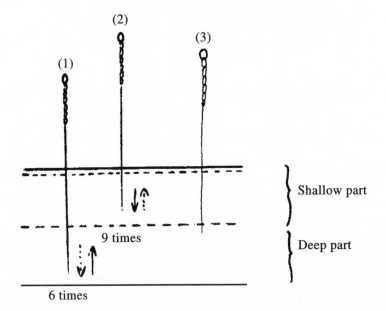

Fig. B-1 Yin concealed Yang method.

C. Dragon Match With Tiger Method

1. Principle:

   The manipulation of tonification and dispersion at the same time based on the twist method is for adjusting nutrient and defensive Qi and to relieve the stagnation of the Qi.

2. Contains: Twist method

3. Indication:

   Various painful disorders, especially intense pain.

4. Method:

   a. The needle is inserted to a certain depth; wait for the arrival of Qi

   b. Rotate the needle based on the twist method nine times for tonification and six times for dispersion.

   Group I: The meridians of L.I., S.I., TW, Sp, Ki, Liv, CV and GV .

      (1) Rotate the needle in a counterclockwise direction for tonification. See Fig. C-1.

      (2) Rotate the needle in a clockwise direction for dispersion. See Fig. C-1

   Group II: The meridians of Lu, Ht, Pc, St, UB and GB

      (1) Rotate the needle in a clockwise direction for tonification. See Fig. C-2.

      (2) Rotate needle in counterclockwise dispersion. See Fig C-2.

   c. Repeat step b if necessary.

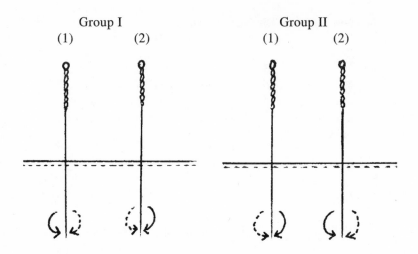

Solid arrow: Forceful rotation
Broken arrow: Gentle rotation

Fig C-1   Fig. C-2

D. Dragon Shaking Tail Method

1. Principle:

   The manipulation of tonification is performed by shaking
   the needle handle to reinforce the movement of the Qi.

2. Indications:

   Deficient syndromes with the stagnation of Qi, Bi-syndrome, indigestion, asthma, PMS.

3. Method:

   a. Insert the needle to a certain depth and wait for or
      hasten the arrival of Qi

   b. Hold the needle handle at an angle with the thumb and
      index finger and direct the point of the needle in the

direction of the diseased area; gently shake the needle handle nine times. See Fig. D-1

c.   Repeat step b several times if necessary.

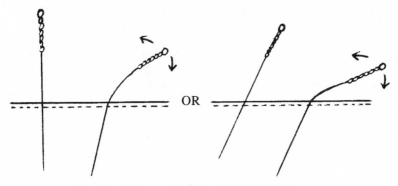

Fig. D-1 Dragon Shaking Tail Method.

E.   Tiger Shaking Head Method

1.   Principle:

The manipulation of dispersion is performed by the twist and lift and thrust methods to relieve stasis of the blood.

2.   Indications:

Excessive syndromes with stasis of the blood such as PMS, physical injuries, amenorrhea, etc.

3.   Method:

a.   Insert the needle to the shallow part of the needle insertion area.

b.   Thrust the needle while at the same time rotating the needle in a counterclockwise direction to the deep part of the needle insertion area. See Fig. E-1.

c.   Lift the needle while at the same time rotating the

needle in a clockwise direction to the shallow part of
the needle insertion area. See Fig. E-1.

d. Shake the needle quickly.

e. Repeat steps b, c and d if necessary.

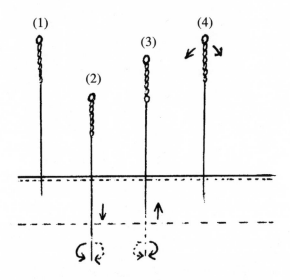

Solid arrow: Forceful movement and rotation
Broken arrow: Gentle movement and rotation
Fig. E-1 Tiger Shaking Head Method

F. The Shao-Shan-Huo Method (Fire of the Volcano Method)

1. Principle:

    The manipulation of the needles in three parts of the
    needle insertion depth to strongly tonify and support the
    Yang Qi and to eliminate Cold Syndromes.

2. Indications:

    Deficient and Cold syndromes of the internal organs,
    deficient and cold syndromes of the stomach or spleen,
    lumbago due to deficiency of kidney, rheumatoid arthritis,

Bi-syndrome, persistent spasm, muscular atrophy, paralysis and irregular menstruation.

3. Method:

a. Determine the depth of insertion and divide it into three parts: the part of sky, of person, and of earth. For example, if 1.5 cun of the depth are to be inserted, the needle will be manipulated between the surface of the body and 0.5 cun and 1.0 cun is the part of person (the deep part); and between 1.0 cun and 1.5 cun is the part of the earth (the deepest part). See Fig. F-1.

b. Ask the patient to take a deep breath and, with the exhalation, insert the needle into the skin and heavily and quickly move the needle down; then gently and slowly move the needle up into the sky part (the shallow part) for nine times. See Fig. F-1.

c. Move the needle down to the part of person; then heavily and quickly move the needle down and gently and slowly move the needle up in this part for nine times. See Fig. F-1.

d. Move the needle down to the part of earth; then heavily and quickly move the needle down and gently and slowly move the needle up in the earth part for nine times. See Fig F-1.

e. Move the needle up to the sky part and repeat steps b, c and d in every ten to fifteen minutes.

f. The needle is withdrawn slowly with the inhalation; press the puncture site gently with a cotton ball after withdrawing the needle.

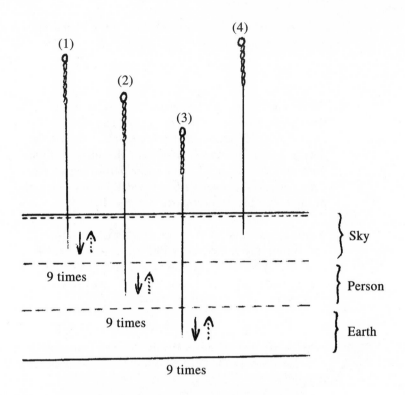

Solid arrow: Heavy and quick movement
Broken arrow: Gentle and slow movement
Fig. F-1 the Shao-Shan-Huo Method.

This method produces a needle sensation that is stronger than other
kinds of tonification methods. Because of this, it is important to pay
attention to the following when applying this method to the patient:

1. Try to avoid applying this method during the patient's first
    treatment. The strong Qi sensation that is elicited could
    give the patient a nervous feeling and this could effect the
    course of the treatment.

2. This method is suitable at points which are located in the
    thicker muscles. Points located on the head, the terminate
    part of the four limbs, and the chest are not suitable for the
    use of this method.

3. Needle manipulation should be applied gently and carefully to patients who are nervous or sensitive to needle sensation.

4. Ask the patient to let you know how the needle sensation feels during needle manipulations so that you can properly adjust the needle manipulation.

5. Apply this method at one or two major points in each treatment.

6. If the patient has no sensation of warm or heat under the needle or through the entire body while using this method, it is advisable to discontinue it. Based on clinical experience, it is difficult to produce warm or heat needle sensations in the following conditions:

   a. extremely deficient syndromes: the needle will feel loose under the skin during needle manipulation.

   b. the patient has a dull needle sensation.

   c. the patient feels too much sharp pain after needle insertion. This will interfere with the needle manipulation making it difficult to produce the warm or heat needle sensation.

G. The Tou-Tien-Liang Method (The cooling of Sky Method)

1. Principle:

   The manipulation of the needles in the three parts of the needle inserting depth to strongly disperse and eliminate the heat syndrome.

2. Indications:

   Febrile and inflammatory disorders, e.g. stomachache, abdominal pain, toothache, swelling pain, tonsillitis and conjunctivitis.

3. Method:

    a. Determine the depth of needle insertion and divide it
        into three parts (sky, person and earth).

    b. Ask the patient to take a deep breath with the inhalation.

    c. Insert the needle into the earth part (the deepest part of
        needle insertion). See Fig G-1.

    d. Gently and slowly move the needle down and heavily
        and quickly move the needle up in this part six times.

    e. Move the needle up to the person part and repeat step d.

    f. Move the needle up to the sky part and repeat step d.

    g. Repeat steps c, d, e and f every ten to fifteen minutes.

    h. The needle is withdrawn quickly with the exhalation
        and the needle hole is kept open.

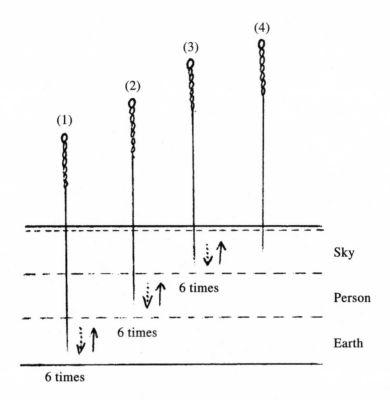

Solid arrow: Heavy and quick movement
Broken arrow: Gentle and slow movement
Fig G-1 Tou-Tien-Liang Method.

This method produces a needle sensation of coolness that is more prominent than with other kinds of dispersion methods. The cautions that apply to the Shao-Shan-Huo Method apply also to this method.

Chapter IV

The Special Techniques for

Even-Tonification and

Even-Dispersion

CHAPTER IV. THE SPECIAL TECHNIQUES FOR EVEN-TONIFICATION AND EVEN-DISPERSION

The techniques of even-tonification and even-dispersion are used in treating conditions which are lacking in clarity in the deficient and excessive syndromes. Various pain disorders and neuralgia. are examples of such conditions. Based on many clinical experiences from ancient times through today, the curative effects are rapid and noteworthy. Clinically, these techniques have been widely performed among acupuncturists throughout the world and great progress has been made in preparing methodology for future use.

A. The Moving Qi Method

1. Principle:

    Induct and move the Qi with both needle manipulation and activity of the affected part of the body to relieve the stagnation of Qi and to balance Yin and Yang.

2. Indications:

    Various pain disorders.

3. Method:

    a. Insert the needle at a certain point located away from the site of the disorder.

    b. Wait for or hasten the arrival of the Qi.

    c. Manipulate the needle after obtaining the Qi and ask the patient to slightly move the affected part of the body.

    d. Repeat step c. every few minutes.

    If the disorder is located in the chest or abdominal area or if the patient has difficulty moving the affected area, massage the affected area before and after manipulation or ask the patient to take a deep breath several times during manipulation. The points used in this method have to be located away from the side of the disorder to make it easy for the patient to activate the affected part and convenient for the practitioner to massage the affected part. The needles are usually inserted in the healthy side of the body. Some specific points are very useful for treating certain disorders, for example, UB 65 is chosen for occipital headache in this method; Sp 4 for frontal headache; GB 31 for migraine headache; Pc 6 for chest fullness or pain; TW 3 for lumbago; S.I. 3 for pain in the knee; TW 6 for pain in the leg; and GB 39 for neck stiffness.

B. The Inverted Horse Method

1. Principle:

The needles are inserted next to each other in the same meridian to reinforce the Qi circulation and enhance the therapeutic effect. This method is associated with the moving Qi method.

2. Indications:

Various disorders, especially for various chronic and persistent diseases.

3. Method:

a. Insert the first needle at a specific point, for example, Pc 6.

b. Insert the second needle next to the first needle in the same meridian, either Pc 5 or Pc 7.

c. Manipulate both needles and ask the patient to slightly move the affected area or apply massage to the affected area before or after manipulating the needles if the affected area is located in the chest or abdominal area, or if the patient can't move the affected area himself.

d. Repeat step c every ten minutes.

There are some recommended specific points that are clinically effective with the use of this method, for example, Pc 5 and Pc 6 for various heart diseases; St 44 and St 45 for various gastro-intestinal disorders; TW 5 and TW 6 for intercostal neuralgia; L.I. 10 and L.I 11 for dizziness, sinusitis, pain in the knee, pain in the arm and shoulder, and lumbago; UB 62 and UB 63 for leg spasm, pain in the head and epilepsy.

C. The Tractive Method

1. Principle:

The manipulation of both a treat point (a remote point located in the healthy side) and a tractive point (a remote point located on the affected side) at the same time for the Qi to tractive each other in those two points and pass through the disorder's area to relieve the painful disorders. This method is associated with the move Qi and inverted horse methods.

2. Indication:

Persistent pain disorders.

3. Method:

a. Insert the first needle in a certain remote point of the healthy side as a treat point, for example, GB 31.

b. Insert the second needle in a certain remote point of the disorder side as a tractive point, for example, TW 5.

c. Manipulate both needles at the same time.

d. Massage the disorder's area before and after manipulating needles.

e.   Repeat steps c and d every ten minutes. If the pain is
     located in the center of the thumb of body, e.g. chest
     pain or abdominal pain, insert needles in the remote
     points of both side (needled bilateral, two treat points
     and two tractive points). Manipulate two needles at the
     same time and all of four needles have to be manipu-
     lated.

This method is easy to operate and often produces a
remarkable result. For instance, in a case of pain in the
lateral part of the elbow of the left arm, insert the first
needle at GB 31 of the right side of body (the healthy side)
as a treat point, and insert second needle at TW 5 of the
left side of body (disorder side) as a tractive point. Manipulate both needles at the same time and massage the
elbow of the left arm before and after manipulation of the
needles.

In a case of pain in the right side of the frontal part of the
shoulder, insert the first needle at St 40 of the left side of
body (healthy side) as a treat point, and insert second
needle at L.I. 4 of the right side of body (disorder side) as
a tractive point. Similarly, for pain in the left side of the
posterior aspect of the knee, insert the first needle at Ht 3
of the right side of body as a treat point, and insert the
second at Ki 3 of the left side of body (disorder side) as a
tractive point.

If the disorder is located in both sides of body, for example, bilateral pain in the posterior part of the knees,
insert two needles at Ht 3 of both sides as a treat point and
insert another needle at Ki 3 of both sides as a tractive
point, then manipulate all four needles (two needles at the
same time) and massage both knees before and after
manipulating needles. The recommended points chosen for
this method are listed in the following table:

Location of disorders	Frontal	Posterior	Lateral
3 Yang-Hands	L.I.	S.I.	TW
3 Yin-Feet	Sp	Ki	Liv
3 Yin-Hands	Lu	Ht	Pc
3 Yang-Feet	St	UB	GB

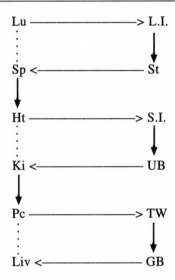

From the above tables, if choosing remote points from the L.I. meridian as a treat or tractive point, another point is chosen from the St meridian as a treat or tractive point, and those of S.I. to UB, TW to GB, Lu to Sp, Ht to Ki, Pc to Liv. The remote points from each group of meridians are chosen based on the location of the disorders, e.g. the remote points from meridians of Lu, Sp, L.I. and St are for the disorders located in the frontal part of body; Ht, Ki, S.I. and UB for the posterior part of the body, and Pc, Liv, TW and GB for the lateral parts of body.

Chapter V

The Point Through to Point

Therapeutics

CHAPTER V.   POINT THROUGH TO POINT
THERAPEUTICS

Point through to point therapeutics is a method in which one needle
is used to needle two points. Some common examples of this are:
TW 23 through to GB 8 for treating persistent migraine headaches;
L.I. 4 through to Pc 8 for numbness or pain in the fingers; and GB 34
through to Sp 9 for persistent pain in the knee. The merits of the
point through to point therapeutics are:

1. it enhances the therapeutic effect

2. it utilizes a minimum of points for treating persistent and
    chronic disorders.

3. it strengthens the effect of needle manipulation.

4. it is easy to remember the point prescription since the
    points are located on the same meridian or on an adjacent
    meridian.

The point through to point therapeutics produces a stronger needle
sensation than that of another therapeutics. Therefore, it is important
to pay attention to the following points when applying this technique:

1. Carefully avoid use in old, weak and easy needle - fainting
    patient, or the patient with extremely deficient syndrome.

2. Gently and slowly move the needle from one point through
    to the second point. If it is difficult to move the needle
    through the two points, the needle should be moved
    backwards (angled or left in place for a few minutes before
    continuing again).

3. Carefully manipulate the needle in areas over important
    organs.

4. After removing the needle, apply pressure with cotton for a
    few seconds to avoid bleeding or hematoma.

5. If the needle is bent, broken, or if the patient has needle-fainting, the management is the same as with routine acupuncture techniques.

A. Fengchi (GB 20) Through To Fengchi (GB 20)

1. Contains: Two Fengchi (GB 20) points.

2. Indications: Headache; pain or stiffness in the neck; eye disorders and mental illness.

3. Method: Insert the needle horizontally 1.5 - 3 cun from GB 20 to the opposite side of GB 20.

4. Needle Sensation: Soreness and distention that spreads over the occipital area of the head and down to the neck

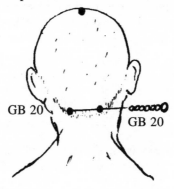

Fig. 1: Fengchi (GB 20) through the Fengchi (GB 20)

B. Yingxiang (L.I. 20) through to Biton

1. Contains: Yingxiang (L.I. 20) and Biton points.

2. Point Location of Biton: Midway between (L.I. 20) and Jingming (UB 1)

3. Indications: Chronic sinusitis.

4. Method: Insert the needle horizontally upward 0.5 - 1 cun from L.I. 20 to Biton.

5. Needle sensation: Distention, pain and tearing of eyes.

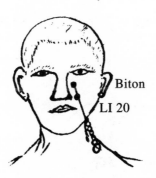

Fig. 2: Yingxiang (L.I. 20) through to Biton

C. Ermen (TW 21) and Xiaguan (St 7) T-needle

1. Contains: Ermen (TW 21), Tingon (S.I. 19), Tinghui (GB 2) and Xiaguan (St 7).

2. Indications: Deafness, heavy hearing and tinnitus.

3. Method:

    a. Insert the first needle horizontally 1 - 1.5 cun along the skin from TW 21 to GB 2.

    b. Insert the second needle horizontally 1 - 1.5 cun along the skin from St 7 to S.I. 19 (pass over S.I 19).

4. Needle sensation: Numbness and distention around the facial area.

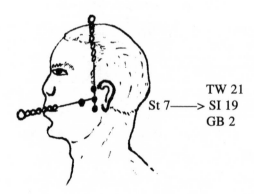

Fig. 3: Ermen (TW 21) and Xiaguan (St 7) T-needle.

D. Zhongwan (CV 12) through to Shanwan (CV 13)

1. Contains: Zhongwan (CV 12) and Shanwan (CV 13).

2. Indications: Chronic stomach and duodenum ulceration; acute and chronic gastritis, gastroptosis; vomiting; diarrhea; constipation; indigestion.

3. Method: Insert 1 - 2 cun horizontally along the skin from Zhongwan (CV 12) to Shanwan (CV 13)

4. Needle Sensation: Distention or heaviness in the upper part of the abdomen with sensation of constriction in the stomach.

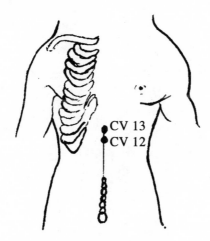

Fig. 4: The Zhongwan (CV 12) through to Shanwan (CV 13)

E. Weishu (UB 21) through to Pishu (UB 20)

1. Contains: Weishu (UB 21) and Pishu (UB 20)

2. Indications: Ulcerations of the stomach and duodenum; gastroptosis; chronic hemorrhagia of the gastrointestine; nervous vomiting; indigestion; hepatomegalia; megalosplenia; pancreatitis; hepatitis.

3. Method: Insert 1.0 - 1.5 cun horizontally along the skin from UB 21 to UB 20.

4. Needle Sensation: Soreness, numbness and distention that spreads over the abdomen.

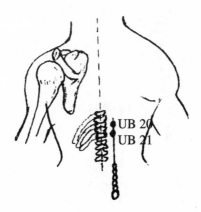

Fig. 5: Weishu (UB 21) through to Pishu (UB 20)

F. The Clear Eyesight Method

1. Contains: Gaohuangshu (UB 43) and Jianzhongshu (S.I 15).

2. Indication: Eye disorders.

3. Method: Insert the needle horizontally along the skin from UB 43 to S.I. 15.

4. Needle Sensation: soreness and numbness spreading to the upper part of the shoulder and upward toward the eyes.

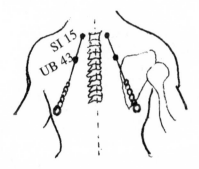

Fig. 6: Gaohuangshu (UB 43) through to Jianzhongshu (S.I. 15)

G. The Dingchuang Method

1. Contains: Yaoshu (GV 2) and Yaoyangguan (GV 3).

2. Indications: Bronchitis; bronchitic asthma; rheumatic lumbago.

3. Method:

    a. Divide the distance from GV 2 to GV 3 into six equal parts.

    b. Insert respectively 7 needles 0.3 - 0.5 cun horizontally along the skin with the needle directed upward.

4. Needle Sensation: numbness, distention and soreness around the lower back area.

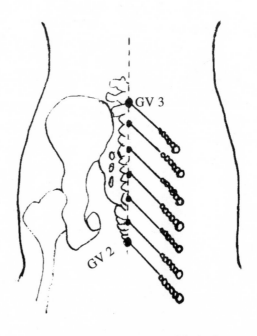

Fig. 7: The Dingchuang Method.

H. The Clear Lung Method

1. Contains: Taiyuan (Lu 9) and Jingqu (Lu 8)

2. Indications: Chronic trachitis.

3. Method: Insert obliquely 1 - 1.5 cun from Lu 9 to Lu 8.

4. Needle Sensation: Soreness, numbness and distention spreading up to the arm and down to the fingers.

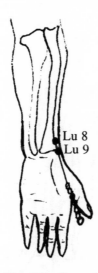

Fig. 8: The Clear Lung Method.

I.   The Strengthen Heart Method

1.   Contains: Daling (Pc 7), Neiguan (Pc 6), Jianshi (Pc 5),
     and Ximen (Pc 4).

2.   Indications: Weakness of the vigor of the mind; poor
     circulation of the terminates; shock; collapse; dizziness;
     hypotension; epilepsy; vomiting; hysteria; tachycardia.

3.   Method: Insert 5.5 cun horizontally from Pc 7 to Pc 4
     along the skin with the needle directed upward.

4.   Needle Sensation: Soreness and numbness spreading up to
     the shoulder and down to the fingers.

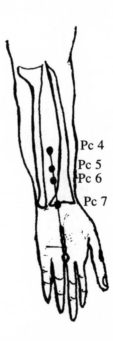

Fig. 9: The strengthen heart method.

J. Hypnotism

1. Contains: Shenmen (Ht 7), Yinxi (Ht 6), Tongli Ht 5) and Lingdao (Ht 4).

2. Indications: Insomnia; epilepsy; mental illness; palpitation; hypertension; hypotension; neurasthenia; hysteria.

3. Method: Insert 2.5 cun horizontally from Ht 7 to Ht 4 along the skin with the needle directed upward.

4. Needle Sensation: Soreness, numbness and distention around the wrist, arm and shoulder.

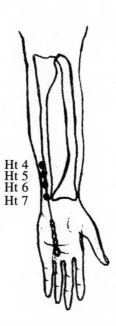

Ht 4
Ht 5
Ht 6
Ht 7

Fig. 10: Hypnotism

K. Neiguan (Pc 6) through to Waiguan (TW5)

1. Contains: Neiguan (Pc 6) and Waiguan (TW 5)

2. Indications: Pain in the joint of the wrist; ringing in the ear; sore throat; hand tremor.

3. Method: Insert 1.0 - 1.5 cun perpendicularly.

4. Needle Sensation: soreness, distention and numbness spreading to the fingers.

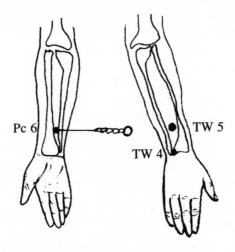

Fig. 11: Neiguan (Pc 6) through to Waiguan (TW 5)

L. Quchi (L.I. 11) and Quze (Pc 3) T-needle

1. Contains: Quchi (L.I. 11), Shaohai (Ht 3), and Quze (Pc 3).

2. Indications: Paralysis of the upper extremities; pain in the joints of the shoulder and elbow; pain and swelling in the pharynx and larynx; fever; goiter; urticaria.

3. Methods:
    a. Insert the first needle 1.5 - 2.5 cun from L.I. 11 to Ht 3
    b. Insert the second needle 1 cun from Pc 3 to Ht 3.

4. Needle sensation: numbness and soreness spreading to wrist or hand.

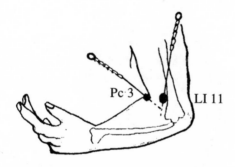

Fig. 12: Quchi (L.I. 11) and Quze (Pc 3) T-needle

M. Hegu (L.I. 4) through to Laogong (Pc 8)

1. Contains: Hegu (L.I. 4) and Laogong (Pc 8)

2. Indications: Hand and foot tremors; polyhydrosis in the hand; hysteria; headache; toothache; hysterical paralysis; mental illness.

3. Method: Insert 1.5 - 2.5 cun obliquely at a 75 degree angle from L.I. 4 to Pc 8.

4. Needle sensation; nunbness and distention spreading to the fingers.

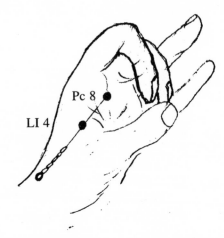

Fig. 13: Hegu (L.I. 4) through to Laogong (Pc 8)

N. Yanglingquan (GB 34) through to Yinglingquan (Sp 9)

1. Contains: Yanglingquan (GB 34) and Yinglingquan (Sp 9).

2. Indications: Pain in the joint of the knee; sciatica; hemiplegia; intercostal neuralgia; constipation; cholecystitis.

3. Method: Insert the needle 2 - 3 cun perpendicularly from GB 34 to Sp 9.

4. Needle Sensation: Soreness and distension toward the lower part of the leg.

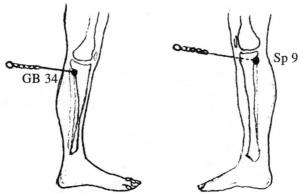

Fig 14: Yanglingquan (GB 34) through to Yinglingquan (Sp 9)

O. Xuanzhong (GB 39) through to Sanyinjiao (Sp 6)

1. Contains: Xuanzhong (GB 39) and Sanyinjiao (Sp 6).

2. Indications: neck stiffnes; pain in the knee and ankle; nephritis.

3. Method: Insert 2.0 - 2.5 cun perpendicularly from GB 39 to Sp 6.

4. Needle sensation: Soreness and distension toward the foot.

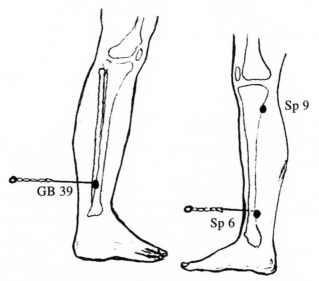

Fig. 15. Xuanzhong (GB 39) through to Sangyinjiao (Sp 6)

P. Huantiao (GB 30) through to Chengfu (UB 50)

1. Contains: Huantiao (GB 30) and Chengfu (UB 50).

2. Indications: Sciatica; lumbago; paralysis in the lower limbs; constipation.

3. Method: Insert 3-4 cun obliquely at 45° from GB 30 to UB 50.

4. Needle sensation: Numbness, soreness and distention aroundthe needle area and spreading down to the leg.

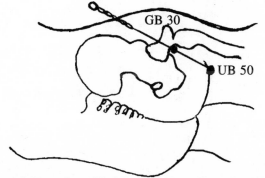

Fig. 16. Huantiao (GB 30) through to Chengfu (UB 50)

Q. Tiokou (St 38) through to Chengshan (UB 57)

1. Contains: Tiaokou (St 38) and Chengshan (UB 57)

2. Indications: Sciatica; hemorrhoids; shoulder pain.

3. Method: Insert 1.5 - 2.0 cun obliquely from St 38 to UB 57.

4. Needle Sensation: Soreness and distention spreading around the leg.

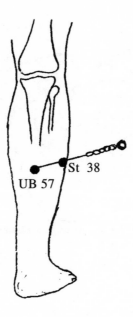

Fig. 17: Tiaokou (St 38) through to Chengshan (UB 57)

R. Kunlun (UB 60) through to Taixi (Ki 3)

1. Contains: Kunlun (UB 60) and Taixi (Ki 3)

2. Indications: Pain in the foot and heel; sciatica; pain in the joint of the ankle; irregular menstruation; toothache; chronic sore throat; ringing in the ear; headache; neck stiffness; pain in the lower part of the back; and paralysis of the lower limbs.

3. Method: Insert 0.5 - 1.0 cun perpendicularly from UB 60 to Ki 3.

4. Needle sensation: soreness and distension around the ankle area and toward the leg.

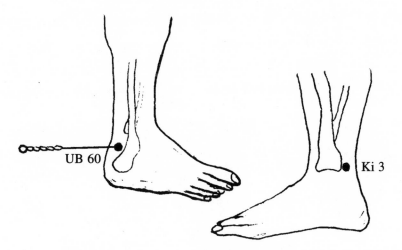

Fig. 18.: Kunlun (UB 60) through to Taixi (Ki 3)

Chapter VI

The Assemble Points Therapeutics

CHAPTER VI. THE ASSEMBLE POINTS THERAPEUTICS

The "Assemble Points Therapeutics" is a method of combining two or more points in a group for enhancing the therapeutic effect. Some example of this method are: Head Tri-needle (consisting of one Yintang point and two Taiyang points) for treating headache and dizziness; hypnotism consists of Shenman (Ht 7), Yinxi (Ht 6), Tonli (Ht 5) and Lingdao (Ht 4) for insomnia, epilepsy, palpitation,neurasthenia, hysteria and mental illness.

The direction of needle insertion in this method is usually horizontal or oblique. The merits of the Assemble Points Therapeutics are a higher curative effect and the use of a minimum of points for treating persistent and chronic disorders.

A. Head Tri-Needle

1. Point Prescription: Taiyang and Yintang points

2. Indications: Headache and dizziness

3. Point location:

    a. Taiyang: 1 finger-breadth posterior to a point midway
        between the lateral extremity of the eyebrow and the
        lateral corner of the eye at the bony edge.

    b. Yintang: between the medial extremities of the
        eyebrows at the midline.

4. Method:

    a. Insert the first two needles obliquely 0.5 - 1.0 cun at
        both Taiyang points

    b. Insert the third needle obliquely 0.5 cun at Yintang
        with the needle directed downward.

5. Needle sensation: Soreness and distention spread around
    the head and facial area.

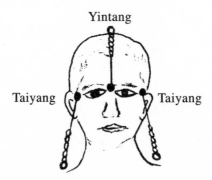

Fig. 1: Head Tri-Needle

B. Neck Tri-Needle

1. Point Prescription: Anmin point, Dazhui (GV 14)

2. Indication: Neurasthenia, insomnia, epilepsy and hysteria

3. Point location:

   Anmin: at the mid-point between Fengchi (GB 20) and Yifeng (TW 17)

4. Method:

   a. Insert the first and second needles obliquely 1.0 cun at Anmin point bilaterally.

   b. Insert the third needle 0.5 - 1.0 cun perpendicularly or obliquely at Dazhui (GV 14).

5. Needle Sensation: distension and spreading to the head and shoulders or toward the lumbar area.

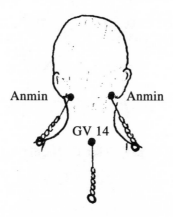

Fig. 2: Neck Tri-Needle.

C. Chest Tri-Needle

1.   Point Prescription: Rugen (St 18), Shanzhong (CV 17)

2.   Indications: Lactation deficiency and mastitis.

3.   Methods.

   a.   Insert the first and second needles obliquely 0.5 cun at both of the Rugen points. There will be a needle sensation of distension around the needled area.

   b.   Insert the third needle 0.5 cun horizontally at CV 17 with the needle directed downward.

4.   Needle Sensation: Distension around the needled area.

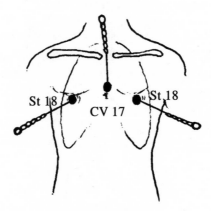

Fig. 3: Chest Tri-Needle.

D. Upper Abdominal Tri-Needle.

1. Point Prescription: Weishan, Zhongwan (CV 12)

2. Indications: upper abdominal pain and gastroptosis.

3. Point location:

    Weishan: 2.0 cun superior to the unbilicus and 4.0 cun
    laterior to the midline of the abdomen.

4. Methods:

    a. Insert the first and second needles 1.0 cun horizontally
        along the skin at both Weishan points with the needles
        angled toward the umbilicus.

    b. Insert the third needle perpendicularly 1.0 - 2.0 cun at
        CV 12.

5. Needle Sensation: soreness, distension and numbess
    around the abdominal area.

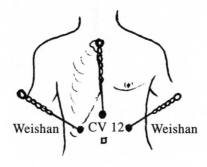

Fig. 4: Upper Abdominal Tri-Needle

E. Umbilical Tri-Needle

1. Point Prescription: Tianshu (St 25), Zhishieh

2. Indications: chronic diarrhea, acute and chronic enteritis and dysentery.

3. Point location: Zhisheih: 2.5 cun inferior to the umbilicus, on the midline of the abdomen.

4. Methods:

    Insert three needles perpendicularly 1.0 -2.0 cun at Tianshu (St 25) and Zhishieh points respectively.

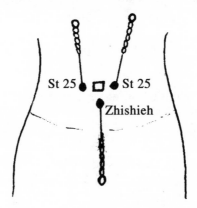

Fig. 5: Umbilical Tri-Needle

F. Lower Abdominal Tri-Needle

1. Point Prescription: Zhongji (CV 3), Zikoun

2. Indications: Seminal emission, impotence, irregular menstruation, leukorrhea, enuresis, retention of the urine, and frequency of micturition.

3. Point location:

    Zikoun: 4.0 cun inferior to the umbilicus and 3.0 cun lateral to the midline of the abdomen.

4. Method: Insert three needles 1.0 - 2.0 cun perpendicularly at Zhongji (CV 3) and Zikoun (2 needles) points respectively.

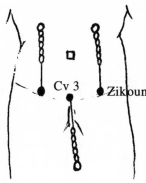

Fig. 6: Lower Abdominal Tri-Needle

G. Plums Tri-Needle

1. Point Prescription: Guanyuan (CV 4), Fukoun.

2. Indications: Infertility, ovarioncus, ovaritis, and testitis.

3. Point location:

   Fukoun: 1.5 cun inferior to the umbilicus and 2.5 cun
   lateral to the midline of the abdomen.

4. Method: Insert three needles 1.0 - 2.0 cun perpendicularly
   at Guanyuan (CV 4) and Fukoun (2 needles) points
   respectively. This has a needle sensation of distension
   around lower part of the abdomen after obtaining the Qi.

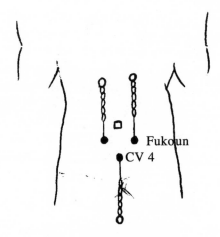

Fig. 7: Plums Tri-Needle

H. Back Tri-Needle

1. Point Prescription: Dazhui (GV 14), Dingchuang

2. Indications: cough, asthma, high fever, and infections in
    the upper respiratory tract.

3. Point Location:

    Dingchuang: 0.5 cun lateral to Dazhui (GV 14).

4. Methods:

    a. Insert the first and second needles 0.5 - 1 cun ob-
        liquely at both of the Dingchuang points with the
        needle directed toward the spinous process.

    b. Insert the third needle 0.5 cun perpendicularly at the
        Dazhui (GV 14).

5. Needle sensation: numbness and distension spreading
    around the neck, head and shoulders.

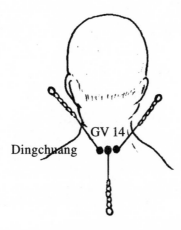

Fig. 8: Back Tri-Needle

I. Lumbar Tri-Needle

1. Contains: Shenshu (UB 23), Mingmen (GV 4)

2. Indications: Lumbago and lumbar sprain.

3. Methods:

    a. Insert the first needle 0.5 - 1.0 cun perpendicularly at
        Mingmen (GV 4).

    b. Insert the second and third needles 1.0 - 1.5 cun
        perpendicularly at both of the Shenshu points.

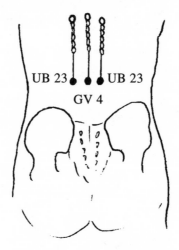

Fig. 9: Lumbar Tri-Needle

J. Shoulder Tri-Needle

1. Point Prescription: Jianyu (L.I. 15), Jianchen, Jianhouh

2. Indications: Persistent pain in the shoulder and upper extremities.

3. Point location:

    a. Jianchen: 1.0 cun superior to the crease of the anterior armpit.

    b. Jianhouh: 1.5 cun superior to the crease of the posterior armpit.

4. Methods:

    a. Insert the first needle 1.0 -3.0 cun obliquely at Jianyu (L.I. 15). The needle is placed against the deltoideus muscle toward the intero-inferior insertion.

    b. Insert the second and third needles 1.5 cun obliquely at the Jianchen and Jianhouh points.

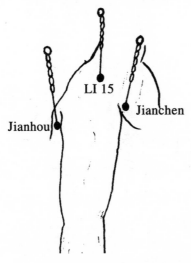

Fig. 10: Shoulder Tri-Needle

K. Hand Tri-Needle

1. Point Prescription: Zhongwan, Chiguan, and Naoguan
    points.

2. Indications: Paralysis in the upper limb, numbness in the
    hand, difficulty in stretching the fingers, and headache.

3. Point Location:

    a. Zhonguan: 1.0 cun superior to the crease of the back
        of the wrist between the radius and ulna.

    b. Chiguan: 1.0 cun superior to the crease of the back of
        the wrist and1 cun lateral to the midline of the anterior
        arm lateral to the ulna.

    c. Naoguan: 1.0 cun superior to the crease of the back of
        the wrist and1.0 cun lateral to the midline of the
        anterior arm lateral to the radius.

4. Method: Insert three needles 1.0 - 2.0 cun horizontally at
    Zhanguan, Chiguan and Naoguan respectively.

5. Needle Sensation: soreness distension and numbness
    around the hand and arm.

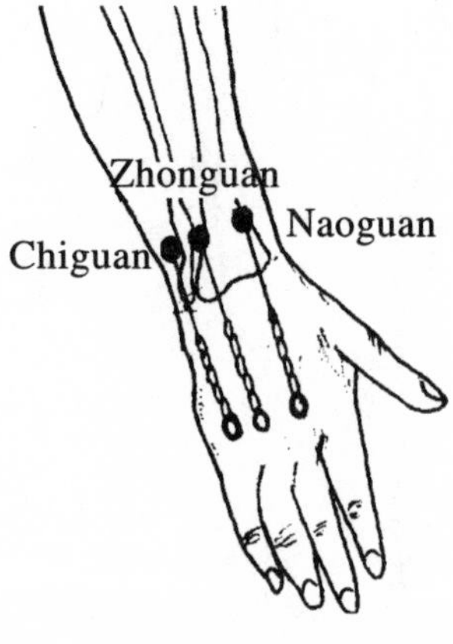

Fig. 11: Hand Tri-Needle

L. Knee Tri-Needle

1. Point Prescription: Dubi (St 35), Yanglingquan (GB 34)

2. Indications: pain in the joint of the knee and knee sprain.

3. Methods:

   a. Insert the first and second needles 1.0 - 2.0 cun obliquely at both Dubi (St 35) points. The needles are to be directed toward the medial part of the knee. The needle sensation is soreness and distension around the knee.

   b. Insert the third needle 1.0 - 2.0 cun perpendicularly at Yanglingquan (GB 34). The needle sensation is numbness and distention that spreads over the leg toward the foot.

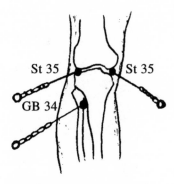

Fig. 12: Knee Tri-Needle

M. Ankle Tri-Needle

1. Point Prescription: Taixi (Ki 3), Kunlun (UB 60), Jiexi (St 41)

2. Indications: Pain in the ankle joint and sprain of the ankle.

3. Method: Insert three needle 0.5 - 1.0 cun perpendicularly at Taixi (Ki 3), Kunlun (UB 60) and Jiexi (St 41) respectively.

4. Needle sensation: distension spreading over the ankle.

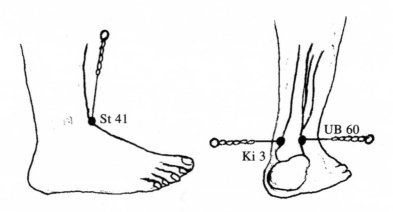

Fig. 13: Ankle Tri-Needle

N. Spinal Tri-Needle

1. Point Prescription: Ji -1, Ji - 2, and Ji - 3 points.

2. Indications: Persistent pain in the back and lumbar area.

3. Point locations:

   a. Ji - 1: 0. 5 cun lateral to the spinous process of the 3rd cervical vertebra.

   b. Ji - 2: 0.5 cun lateral to the spinous process of the 2nd thoracic vertebra.

   c. Ji - 3: 0.5 cun lateral to the spinous process of the 5th lumbar vertebra.

4. Method: Insert 1.0 - 1.5 cun obliquely with the needle toward the vertebra.

5. Needle sensation: distension

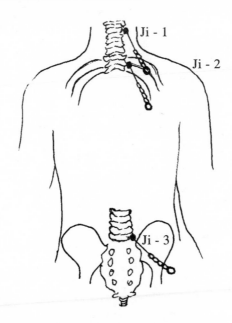

Fig. 14: Spinal Tri-Needle

Chapter VI

Acupuncture Technique

for an Emergency

CHAPTER VII. ACUPUNCTURE TECHNIQUES FOR AN EMERGENCY

In certain conditions, acupuncture techniques for an emergency are more economical, convenient and without side-effects as compared to herbal therapeutics. Over the past 300 years, acupuncture in China has developed various techniques based on extensive and valuable clinical experience in the treatment of medical emergencies with remarkable results.

A. Shock

In Chinese medical science, shock is the manifestation of an imbalance of Yin and Yang and the disturbance of Qi and Blood. The clinical signs include coolness in the four limbs, low blood pressure, cold sweating and, in severe cases, coma. The purpose of acupuncture treatment is to raise the blood pressure, warm the meridians, re-establish the Yang Qi and adjust the function of the Qi and Blood

1. Mild case: The use of needles is not necessary. Pinching or pressing heavily with the finger at Renzhong (GV 26) will revive the patient.

2. Severe Case:

    a. Insert the first needle obliquely upward 0.3 - 0.5 cun at GV 26.

    b. Insert the second and third needles perpendicularly 0.3 - 0.5 cun at Yongquan (Ki 1) and Baihui (GV 20).

The points GV 20, GV 26 and Ki 1 are called the Three Talented Points and are very suitable for emergency situations.

    c. Apply moxa stick over GV 20, CV 8, and CV 4.

B. Heart Attack

1. Insert needles bilateraly at Zusanli (St 36). The manipula-
    tion method to be applied at those two points is dispersion.

2. Insert needles at Neiguan (Pc 6) and Shenmen (Ht 7) if the
    patient has the symptom of tachycardia.

3. Insert needles at Hegu (L.I.4) if the patient has the symp-
    tom of dyspnea.

The purpose of using a dispersion technique at St 36 is for the effect
of sedation; the combination of Pc 6 and Ht 7 has a sedative effect
and strengthens heart function.

C. Stroke (CVA - Cardiovascular Accident)

There are two different kinds of stroke in Chinese medical science:
tense (excessive) syndrome and flaccid (deficient) syndrome. The
clinical signs of a tense syndrome are retention of urine, coarse breathing, redness of the face and ears, a tight closed mouth, coma and a
forceful and wiry pulse. In a flaccid syndrome, the symptoms include
incontinence of urine, cold limbs, sweat over the hands and face, coma,
and a weak and forceless pulse.

Method:

1. Tense (excessive) Syndrome

    a. Bloodletting at Shixuan or Shijing Points (Fig. 1).

    b. Insert needles at Hegu (L.I. 4), Zusanli (St 36),
        Xiaguan (St 7) Zhongji (CV 3) and Taichun (Liv 3) for
        dispersion.

    c. Apply moxa stick over Guanyuan (CV 4), Qihai (CV
        6) and Yangquan (Ki 1).

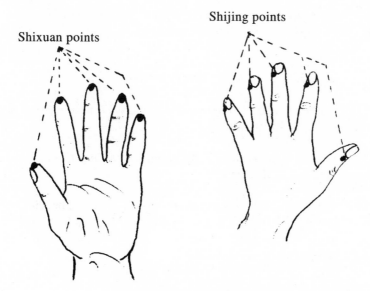

Fig. 1: Shixuan and Shijing Points

2. Flaccid (deficient) Syndrome

    a.   Inset needles at Renzhong (GV 26), Hegu (L.I. 4),
         Neiguan (Pc 6) and Zusanli (St 36) for tonification.

    b.   Apply moxa stick over GV 20, CV 4 and CV 8.

D. Various Acute Hemorrhages

The Xi (cleft) Points of the 12 meridians (Lu 6, Ht 6, Pc 4, L.I. 7, S.I. 6, TW 7, Sp 8, Ki 5, Liv 6, St 34, UB 63 and GB 36) are chosen for the treatment of various acute hemorrhages based on the involved organs and meridians. In addition to Xi Points, Sanyinjiao(Sp 6), Yinbai (Sp 1), Dadun (Liv 1) and Baihui (GV 20) work together to treat various acute hemorrhages. Clinically, the causative factor of the hemorrhage must be determined and surgery may be required as a supplement. Menorrhagia is one of the most commonly treated disorders in the category of acupuncture treatment for emergency. The following prescription has been widely used and has a great remarkable effect: insert needles bilaterally at Sp 6, CV 4 and GV 20; next, apply moxa stick over GV 20, Sp 1 and Liv 1.

E. Acute Asthma Attack (Bronchial Asthma)

1. Insert a needle obliquely 1–2 cun at CV 17; needle points CV 4, St 40, and Lu 5.

2. Insert 0.5 cun needles in the ear points of Pingchuan Shenmen and Lung area.

3. When the crisis of acute attack is over, insert the needles perpendicularly at UB 13, UB 15, UB 23 (bilaterally) and at GV 4 or at points chosen according to the presenting symptoms.

F. Acute Gastroenteritis

The major symptoms of this condition are vomiting and diarrhea. It usually results from eating contanimated food. The treatment is to insert needles at Zhongwan (CV 12), Zusanli (St 36), Tianshu (St 25) and Guanyuan (CV 4). The needles should be retained in place for a longer period of time and manipulated frequently. If the patient has severe vomiting, insert needles at Neiguan (Pc 6). If the patient has low blood pressure, apply moxa stick over Shenque (CV 8) exception to above needled points. Bloodletting at Weizhong (UB 54) and Chize (Lu 5) is applicable. Give warm water with a small amount of salt if the patient is dehydrated.

G. Acute Diarrhea

Insert needle in Quchi (L.I. 11), Shangjuxu (St 37), Zhangwan (CV 12) and Zusanli (St 36). If the patient has a high fever, Hegu (L.I. 4) is chosen; Tianshu (St 25) is selected for the treatment of abdominal pain. The needle manipulation at the above points should result in a strong stimulation and the needles should be retained in place for a longer period of time.

H. Retention of Urine

The symptom of retention or urine can be present in a number of disorders. The following acupuncture treatment for use in this case has a remarkable effect: insert needles at Zhongji (CV 3), Yinlingquan (Sp 9), Guanyuan (CV 4) and Zusanli (St 36). Needle manipulation at the above points should get a strong stimulus, especially at CV 3 and Sp 9 where the needle sensation should spread toward the urinary bladder.

I. High Fever

For the treatment of a high fever, bloodletting at Sansun Points (Fig. 2), is effective. Insert a needle at Dazhui (GV 14). Needling Hegu (L.I. 4) and Quchi (L.I. 11) is applicable if the fever is persistent.

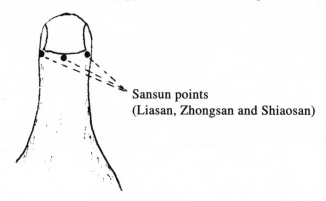

Sansun points
(Liasan, Zhongsan and Shiaosan)

Fig 2: Sansun Points

J. Allergic Itching

Insert needles at Quchi (L.I. 11), Xuihai (Sp 10) and Sanyinjiao (Sp 6) and apply a strong dispersion technique of needle manipulation. Bloodletting at Weizhong (UB 54) is applicable.

K. Acute Stomachache

Insert needles at Liangqui (St 34), Zusanli (St 36) and Zhongwan (CV 12). If the patient has the symptom of vomiting, Neiguan (Pc 6) is chosen; Tianshu (St 25) is chosen for diarrhea.

L. Acute Tonsillitis

The clinical signs of acute tonsillitis are fever, sore throat, dysphagia and swollen tonsils. The treatment is to insert needles at Hegu (L.I. 4) followed by bloodletting at Shaoshang (Lu 11) and Shangyang (L.I. 1). The needle manipulation at these points has to be a strong disperson technique.

M. Acute Toothache

1. Insert needles to a depth of 1.0 - 1.5 cun perpendicularly at L.I. 4.

2. Insert needles to a depth of 1.5 cun obliquely at St 36.

3. Insert needles to a depth of 0.5 - 1.0 cun perpendicularly at St 41 and St 44.

N. Conjunctivitis

1. Bloodletting at UB 15, UB 18 and St 36.

2. Insert needles to a depth of 0.5 cun obliquely at UB 1, UB 2 and Liv 3.

3. Insert needles to a depth of 1.0 - 1.5 cun perpendicularly at L.I.4

O. Alcohol Intoxication

Insert a needle to a depth of 0.5 cun obliquely or perpendicularly at

GV 25 and apply a strongly stimulate for dispersing the stasis of blood in the head and the flare-up of heat from the stomach and spleen.

P.   Acute Intercostal Neuralgia

Insert needles at GB 34 and TW 6 and apply the "Move Qi" method (see page 261) to manipulate needles.

Q. Acute Lumbago

1.   Bloodletting at UB 54

2.   Insert needles to a depth of 0.5 - 1.0 cun at S.I. 3.

3.   Insert neeldes to a depth of 1.0 - 1.5 cun at UB 23.

4.   Insert needles to a depth of 2.0 - 3.0 cun at GB 30.

Apply the "Move Qi" method of manipulation to the above points (see page 261).

R.   Various Acute Sprains

The Move Qi and Tractive Methods of needle manpulation (see pages 261 and 263) are usually used in the following cases:

1.   Acute neck stiffness

   Insert needles at Houxi (S.I. 3) and Xuanzhong (GB 39).

2.   Acute ankle sprain

   Insert needles at Jiexi (St 41), Taixi (Ki 3) and Kunlun (UB 60). Apply the Move Qi Method.

3.   Acute knee joint sprain

   a.   Insert needles at Weizhong (UB 54), Yanglingquan

(GB 34) and Neiguan (Pc 6). Apply the Move Qi
Method.

    b.   Bloodletting at Gaohuang (UB 38).

4.   Acute shoulder joint sprain

    a.   Insert needles at Yanglingquan (GB 34) on the healthy
side as the treatment point.

    b.   Select another point based on the principle of the
Tractive Method as the tractive point (see page 263).

    c.   Apply the Tractive Method (see page 263) to treat this
case.

5.   Acute wrist joint sprain

    a.   Insert a needle at Yanglingquan (GB 34) on the healthy
side.

    b.   Insert another needle at the Ahshi point (tender spot)
on the side of the wrist joint sprain.

Chapter VIII

Practical Electro-Acupuncture

CHAPTER VIII: PRACTICAL ELECTRO-ACUPUNCTURE

Though the history of acupuncture dates back well over 3,000 years, the history of electro-acupuncture is only 40 years old. A relatively new technique, electro-acupuncture is popular all over the world. The purpose and effective use of electro-acupuncture techniques for different kinds of disorders will be examined in this chapter.

A. The Effects of Electro-Acupuncture Stimulation on the Nervous System

It is known that the electric current from the electro-acupuncture machine affects the nervous system, and lower levels of electrical current function in both stimulation and inhibition. When the stimulator is connected to the needles, the afferent nerve located at the puncture site produces a physiological stimulus that is quickly transferred to a specific part of the brain and becomes a prominent electro-cerebral wave. This kind of wave causes either a feeling of sedation much like a light sleep, or a feeling of excitation, depending on the type of electrical wave from the stimulator.

The basic intensity of the stimulation to the nerves and muscles is 35 volts of electric current (3 - 12 Å) with a frequency of 100 cycles per second. A higher level of intensity is needed to treat syndromes of paralysis or muscular atrophy in order to produce muscle contraction and nerve activity. If the patient is especially sensitive to the electric current, he will feel an electric sensation at a low level of intensity. Thus, the degree of intensity of stimulation given to the patient is based on the body constitution of the patient as well as the function of the nervous system, the hematopoietic, circulatory, digestive, urological and endocrine systems.

B. The Functions of the Various Waves of Stimulation

1. Adjustable Wave (Continuous Wave)

The frequency range of the Adjustable Wave is 1–250 cycles per second (c/s). There are two different kinds of adjustable waves:

a.   Dense Wave ($\wedge\!\wedge\!\wedge\!\wedge\!\wedge\!\wedge\!\wedge\!\wedge$)

The frequency range of the Dense Wave is 50 - 250 c/s. It is called the predecessor of the wave because it is used for three to five minutes before other waves are applied in treatment. This wave has the ability to inhibit the function of nervous system response and thus it functions in relieving pain. The body adapts to this wave so the pain relief is only temporary. The clinical function of the dense wave is as follows:

1)   temporary relief of pain

2)   muscle spasm

3)   poor blood circulation due to spasm of the vessels

4)   nervousness

5)   anesthesia

b.   Disperse Wave ($\wedge\!\!\!\!\!\sim\!\!\!\sim\!\!\sim\!\!\vee$)

The frequency range of the Disperse Wave is 1 - 50 c/s. The stimulation that is produced by this wave is stronger than that of the dense wave. Consequently, the patient feels more of a vibrating sensation than with the dense wave. The body does not easily adapt to this wave because the gap of time between the wave is larger than with the Dense wave. The clinical function of this wave is as follows:

1)   Excitation of muscle tissue (effective for syndromes of muscle paralysis).

2)   Stimulation of the growth of connective tissue (effective for tendon injury).

2. Dense-Disperse Wave (〰〰〰〰)

The Dense-disperse wave is one of alternating dense and disperse waves. The body does not adapt to this wave because the gap between the two different kinds of waves is very large. Thus, the dense-disperse wave can be applied for a longer period of time during treatment. The clinical function of the dense-disperse wave is as follows:

a. Strengthen the metabolism (the function of the internal organs).

b. Strengthen blood circulation.

c. Relieve edema due to Bi-syndrome, diabetes and other functional disorders.

d. Pain relief that is effective over a longer period of time

e. Hypertension

f. Muscular disability

g. Arthritis

h. Pain due to sprain

3. Discontinuous Wave (〰〰〰)

The discontinuous wave consists of many dense waves. The vibrating sensation of this wave is the strongest as compared to other kinds of waves and it produces both a very strong needle sensation and muscle contraction response. The clinical function of this wave is as follows:

a. Various types of paralysis

b. Vessel spasm

c. Insomnia

d. Dysmenorrhea

C. The Techniques of Therapeutics

1. The selection of points for stimulation.

    a. Major points: The most effective points for treatment
        of the syndrome or disease are chosen, for example, St
        6 and St 7 for facial paralysis; St 36, CV 12 and Pc 6
        for epigastric pain; L.I. 4 and St 44 for diarrhea due to
        damp-heat.

    b. Tender spot (Ahshi point): The Ahshi point is the
        pressure point, or sensitive point, in acupuncture. It
        could be located in a distal area and be connected to
        the disorder through related meridians.

2. The selection of the electrode.

    The negative electrode is connected to the major point, or
    tender spot, and the positive electrode is connected to a
    subordinate point. Therefore, the negative wire and the
    positive wire must be identified before use in treatment.
    The negative electrode produces a stronger needle sensa-
    tion than the positive electrode. When the electric wires
    are connected to the needles and stimulation applied, the
    patient can identify the negative wire by the strength of
    stimulation.

3. The intensity of stimulation

    The intensity of the vibrating sensation of electro- acu-
    puncture is divided into three different levels. It is based
    on the condition of the disease, the duration of the disease
    and the patient's tolerance to the electric sensation.

    a. Strong: the degree of stimulation is greater than the
        degree of pain; the vibrating sensation is strong.

    b. Moderate: the degree of stimulation causes the muscle
        to contract but the vibrating sensation is comfortable.

    c. Weak: the degree of stimulation is mild; the patient
        may or may not feel the vibrating sensation.

4. The length of time of stimulation per treatment.

    The duration of stimulation is determined by the different types of waves. The general guidelines are:

    a. Dense wave: 5 - 10 minutes

    b. Dense-disperse wave: 10-15 minutes

    c. Discontinuous wave: 15-20 minutes

5. The duration of the therapeutics

    Electro-acupuncture may be applied five to eight times if treatment is given once a day or every other day. This should be followed by a week without electro-acupuncture after which another series of five to eight treatments could be given for a second course if necessary. There is no time limitation if electro-acupuncture is used on a weekly basis.

6. Precautions for the use of electro-acupuncture

    a. The stimulator must be kept in a stable place (to avoid shaking of the unit) and protected from exposure to moisture and high temperatures.

    b. The stimulator must be operated in the recommended manner and its therapeutic function must be applied correctly.

    c. Identify the negative electric wire by needling a few sensitive points and applying stimulation: the stronger vibrating sensation is the negative electrode and the weaker vibrating sensation is the positive electrode.

    d. Do not insert the needles too deeply when they are connected to the stimulator.

    e. Do not connect two wires to one needle.

    f. Check that each output is on the "0" setting before turning on the switch.

7. Contraindications for the use of electro-acupuncture
    treatment

    a. coma

    b. severe heart failure

    c. open type of tuberculosis

    d. malignant tumor

    e. an extremely deficient physical condition

    f. pregnancy

    g. the patient is needle-shy or prone to fainting from
        contact with needles

    h. artificial instrument within the body

Chapter IX

Practical Scalp Acupuncture

Therapeutics

CHAPTER IX: PRACTICAL SCALP ACUPUNCTURE
THERAPEUTICS

Scalp acupuncture therapeutics is a relatively new technique that is
based on a combination of two theories: the theory of channels and
collaterals of Chinese Medical science, and the contemporary medical theory of the functionally fixed location of the cerebricortex (the
outtermost surface of the brain). This technique addresses the treatment of various chronic and systemic disorders. The history of scalp
acupuncture therapeutics is very recent, however there has been a
great deal of clinical research and experience in China as to indicate
that its therapeutic effects are rapid and noteworthy. These remarkable results have stimulated increasing interest among acupuncturists throughout the world.

A. The Anatomy of the Scalp (See Fig. A-1)

The scalp is a soft tissue covering most of the skull. Another soft
tissue covering the skull is the flat musculi capitis. The scalp is divided into six layers as follows:

1. Epidermis: This is the upper layer composed of thick,
    keratin packed cells without nuclei. This layer functions in
    protecting deeper tissue from injury and contains nerves to
    record the conditions of the external environment.

2. Dermis: The dermis contains sebaceous glands which
    provide an oil component for the bacterial flora that
    prevent dryness. Heat regulation is one of the functions in
    this layer.

3. Subcutaneous: The subcutaneous layer varies greatly in
    thickness over different areas of the body. This layer is
    composed of fatty connective tissue. The major blood
    vessels and nerves in the scalp have most of their distribu-
    tion in this layer. The functions of this layer are to insulate
    underlying tissues from extremes of environmental heat or
    cold, as well as to provide a substantial cushion, and to
    provide sensory input of many forms from the body
    surface.

4. Musculus epicranius: This is composed of multiple bundles of fibers to provide a stable base.

5. Epicranial Aponeurosis: This layer is composed of resilient fibers and connects to the flat musculus epicranius and cover the top of the skull.

6. Periosteum: The periosteum is a specialized form of connective tissue. This layer is quite thick in the growing child. As the aging process occurs, it becomes thinner, but is never completely abolished. The function of this layer is to provide for bone growth and remodeling.

The layers of epidermis, dermis and subcutaneous are closely connected to each other. The insertion of needles throughout these three layers will produce a prominent painful feeling and it is difficult to keep the needle in these three layers. Thus, the needle has to be directly inserted into the layer of the epicranial aponeurosis. There are many blood vessels that are distributed in the subcutaneous layer of scalp and the walls of the blood vessels and fibers are close to each other. The blood vessels do not readily contract after needle injury, so bleeding is more likely to occur with acupuncture to the scalp than in the body.

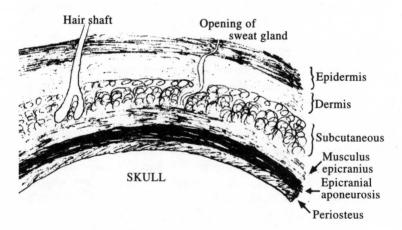

Figure A-1. The Anatomy of the Scalp

B.   The Anatomy of the Skull (Fig. B-1 and B-2)

The skull is composed of a series of flat, irregular bones, which are divided into two categories: the cranium, which protects the brain and which consists of eight bones, and the skeleton of the face, which includes fourteen bones.

The cranium consists of the frontal, occipital, sphenoid, ethmoid, two parietal, and two temporal bones. The following is a lateral view of the skull:

1.   The frontal bone forms the anterior wall.

2.   The occipital bone forms the posterior wall.

3.   The parietal bones form the superior lateral walls.

4.   The temporal bones form the lower lateral walls.

5.   The sphenoid bone forms the floor of the cranial vault, joining anteriorly with the frontal bone and posteriorly with the occipital bone.

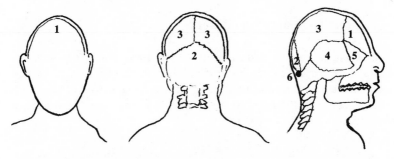

Fig. B-1: The Anterior, Posterior and Lateral Views of the Skull.

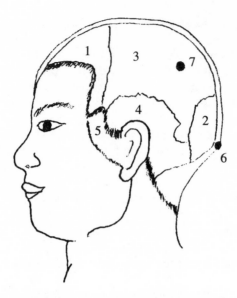

1. frontal bone   2. occipital bone 3. parietal bone
4. temporal bone 5. sphenoid bone
6. exterior occipital protuberance   7. parietal node.

Fig. B-2: The Lateral View of the Skull

C. Gross Anatomy of the Brain

The brain can be divided into three major parts: the brain stem, the cerebellum, and the cerebrum. The brain stem can be sub-divided into medulla, pons, and midbrain. The medulla is part of the brain which connects the brain to the spinal cord. The pons and midbrain are successively more rostra.

1. Cerebrum: The cerebrum is responsible for the highest mental function. It is subdivided into four lobes each of which has special functions. The frontal lobes are in the most anterior part of the cerebrum; the parietal are next to the frontal lobe; the most posterior lobes are the occipital lobes. The temporal lobe is just above the ear.

2. Cerebellum: The cerebellum is located in the angle between the brain stem and the cerebrum. The important

function of the cerebellum is the coordination of motor movement of the muscle.

3. Brain stem: Most of the cranial nerves come from the brain stem. It is the only major pathway between the spinal cord and the higher parts of the brain. The brain stem is especially important in the control of subconscious and reflexive activities such as breathing, heart rate and blood pressure.

D. Functional Anatomy of the Brain (Fig. D-1)

1. Frontal lobe: these are important in two major areas:

    a. Prefrontal cortex: the anterior portion of the frontal lobe. This is especially important in the highest of mental function and in the determination of personality.

    b. Motor cortex: the posterior part of the frontal lobe controls motor movement and modifies movement.

2. Occipital lobe: the occipital lobe is concerned with vision and the recognition of size, shape and color.

3. Temporal lobe: the temporal lobe governs numerous important functions such as behavior and speech.

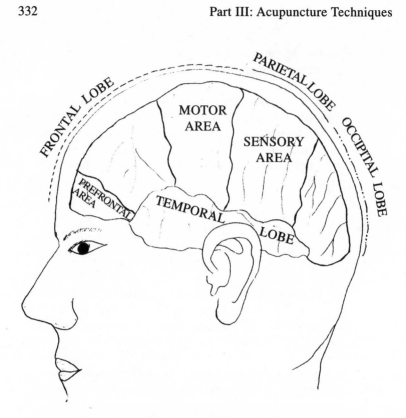

Fig. D-1: The Distribution of the Lobes of the Brain

E. The Cranial Nerves

There are twelve nerves with distribution on the cranial areas:

1. Olfactory nerve (1st cranial nerve): This is the pathway taken by olfactory impulses from the nasal mucosa to the brain.

2. Optic nerve (2nd cranial nerve): This carries information from the eyes for vision and ocular reflexes.

3. Oculomotor Nerve (3rd cranial nerve): This supplies all the intrinsic occular muscles and all extrinsic ocular muscles except for the lateral rectus and superior oblique.

4. Trochlear nerve (4th cranial nerve): This supplies only the superior oblique muscle of the eye.

5. Trigeminal nerve (5th cranial nerve): This is the largest cranial nerve, and it carries fibers that give sensation to the face.

6. Abducent nerve (6th cranial nerve): This supplies the lateral rectus muscle of the eyeball.

7. Facial nerve (7th cranial nerve): This supplies the superficial muscles of the scalp face, and neck and for supply of the lacrimal and salivary glands.

8. Auditory nerve (8th cranial nerve): This is entirely sensory and consists of vestibular and cochlear divisions.

9. Glossopharyngeal nerve (9th cranial nerve): This is a mixed nerve consisting of an afferent part. It supplies the pharynx and tongue, the carotid sinus and body, and the stylopharyngeous muscle.

10. Vagus nerve (10th cranial nerve): This is also a mixed nerve, and it supplies different fibers to the pharynx, esophagus, stomach, larynx, trachea and lungs.

11. Accessory nerve (11th cranial nerve): This consists of bulbar and spinal portions, and controls motor function of the sternomastoid and the trapezius muscles.

12. Hypoglossal nerve (12th cranial nerve): This supplies all the muscles of the tongue.

F. The Location and Indications of the Region of Stimulation in Scalp Acupuncture

The following two "mark" lines will help you to locate the stimulation regions for scalp acupuncture:

> Anterior–posterior middle line: the midpoint of the distance between the eyebrows to the inferior edge of the exterior occipital protuberance of the head.

> Eyebrow–occipital line: the midpoint of the distance between the superior edge of the eyebrow to the apex of the exterior occipital protuberance of the lateral side of the head.

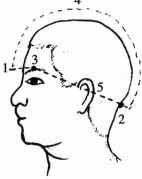

1. The midpoint between the eyebrows
2. Exterior occipital protuberance
3. The midpoint of the superior edge of the eyebrow
4. Anterior–posterior middle line
5. Eyebrow–occipital line

Fig. F–1 The "mark" lines of scalp acupuncture

1. Motor Region

a.   Location: The upper point is located 0.5 cm posterior
to the midpoint of the anterior–posterior middle line.
The lower point is located 0.5 cm anterior to the
junction of the eyebrow–occipital line and a vertical
line at the midpoint of the zygomatic arch (Fig. F–2).
The upper fifth of the motor region is the region of the
lower limbs and trunk; the middle two fifths of the
motor region is the region of the upper limbs; the
lower two fifths of the motor region is the facial
region of the speech region.

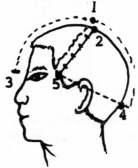

1.   Midpoint of the anterior–posterior middle line
2.   The upper point of the motor region
3.   The midpoint between the eyebrows
4.   Exterior occipital protuberance
5.   The lower point of the motor region

Fig. F–2. The motor region

b.   Indications

1)   Upper 1/5 of the motor region: paralysis of the opposite side of the lower limbs.

2)   Middle 2/5 of the motor region: paralysis of the opposite side of the upper limbs.

3)   Lower 2/5 of the motor region (first speech region): paralysis of the opposite side of the face; speech disorders.

2. Sensory region

    a. Location: 1.5 cm posterior to and parallel with the motor region (Fig. F–3)

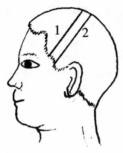 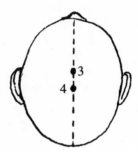

    1. The motor region
    2. The sensory region
    3. The upper point of the motor region
    4. The upper point of the sensory region

Fig. F–3 The sensory region and the upper points of the motor and sensory regions in the parietal part of the head.

    b. Indications

        1) The upper 1/5 of the sensory region: pain and numbness in the opposite side of the lumbar and leg; occipital headache; neck and shoulder pain.

        2) Middle 2/5 of the sensory region: pain and numbness in the opposite side of the upper limbs.

        3) Lower 2/5 of the sensory region: numbness; migraine headache; trigeminal neuralgia; toothache; arthritis in the opposite side of the facial area.

The sensory region combines with corresponding regions (chest, stomach and genital regions) for use in anesthesia for surgery in the corresponding part of the body.

3. Foot motor–sensate region

a. Location: The foot motor sensate region is a straight line 3 cm in length. It is located one cm. lateral to the upper points of the motor and sensory regions and parallel with the anterior–posterior midline (Fig. F–4).

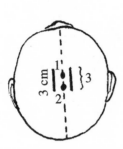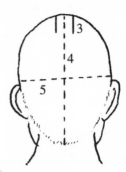

1. The upper point of the motor region
2. The upper point of the sensory region
3. The foot motor sensate region
4. The anterior–posterior middle line
5. Eyebrow–occipital line

Fig. F–4. The parietal and posterior views of stimulate regions

b. Indications

1) Pain, numbness and paralysis in the opposite side of the lumbar area.

2) Insert needles bilaterally for nocturnal enuresis, polyuria and difficult urination.

3) Needle bilaterally and combine with genital region (bilaterally) for polyuria due to acute cyctitis; thirst and polyuria due to diabetes; impotence and seminal emission.

4) Needle bilaterally and combine with intestinal region (bilaterally) for allergic collitis or diarrhea.

5) Needle bilaterally and combine with middle two-fifths of sensory region (bilaterally) for various dermatitis.

4. Chorea-tremor controlled region

a. Location: 1.5 cm anterior to and parallel with motor region (Fig. F–5).

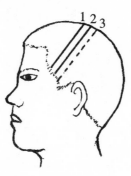

1. Chorea–tremor controlled region
2. Motor region
3. Sensory region

Fig. F–5. The lateral view of stimulate regions

b. Indications

Paralysis agitans; paralysis agitans juvenile; infantile chorea; Parkinson's syndrome.

Insert the needle lateral to the region on the opposite side of the disorder, and bilaterally for symptoms that affect both sides of the body.

5. Vasomotor region

   a. Location: 3 cm. anterior to and parallel with the motor region, or 1.5 cm. anterior to and parallel with the chorea-tremor controlled region (Fig. F–6).

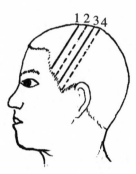

   1. Vasomotor region
   2. Chorea–tremor controlled region
   3. Motor region
   4. Sensory region

Fig. F–6. The lateral view of stimulate regions

   b. Indications

        Cortical edema (edema not due to a dysfunction of the internal organs but from the dysfunction of the cortex [the outermost surface of the brain]). The upper half of the vasomotor region is for treatment of cortical edema in the opposite side of the upper limbs; the lower half of the vasomotor region is for cortical edema in the opposite side of the lower limbs.

6. **Dizziness–hearing region**

    a. Location: This region is 4 cm. in length. The midpoint
of this line is located 1.5 cm. superior to the apex of
the auricle (Fig. F–7).

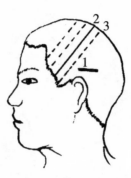

    1. Dizziness–hearing region
    2. Motor region
    3. Sensory region

Fig. F–7. The lateral view of stimulate regions

    b. Indications
        For treatment of tinnitus, Mernier's syndrome and
declining hearing ability, needle on the affected side.
Needle bilaterally for dizziness and motorial epilepsy.

7. **Visual region**

   a. Location: This region is 4 cm. in length. The termina-
       tion of the vertical lines are located on the horizontal
       level of the exterior occipital protuberance and 1 cm.
       lateral to and parallel with the anterior–posterior
       middle line (Fig. F–8).

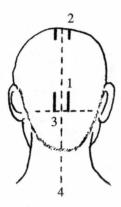

   1. Visual region
   2. Foot motor-sensate region
   3. Horizontal level of the exterior occipital protuberance
   4. Anterior–posterior middle line

   Fig. F–8. The Posterior view of stimulate regions

   b. Indications: Cortical cataract

8. Second speech region

a. Location: The second speech region is 3 cm. in length.
The top of the line is 2 cm. inferior to the parietal
mode, and the line is parallel with anterior–posterior
middle line (Fig. F–9).

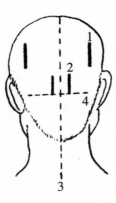

1. Second speech region
2. Visual region
3. Anterior–posterior middle line
4. Horizontal level

Fig. F–9. The posterior view of stimulate regions

b. Indications

Name aphasia (loss of the ability to name an object,
e.g., the patient asking for a pen can only say "to
use for writing").

9. Third speech region

a. Location: The third speech region is 4 cm. in length. The line starts at the mid-point of the dizziness–hearing region (1.5 cm. superior to auricular apex) and stretches 4 cm. toward the occipital area (Fig. F–10).

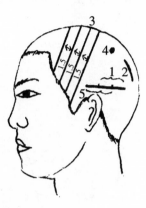

1. Third speech region
2. Second speech region
3. Motor region
4. Parietal node
5. Dizziness–hearing region

Fig. F–10. The lateral view of the stimulate regions

b. Indications

Sensory aphasia (the loss of the ability to understand language and to speak normally; people cannot understand what the patient is saying).

10. Praxia region

a. Location: The praxia region consists of three lines that
    are 3 cm. in length. The first line starts at the parietal
    node and stretches 3 cm. in a vertical line; the second
    and third lines stretch 3 cm. down from the parietal
    node with the first line at a 40 degree angle
    (Fig. F–11).

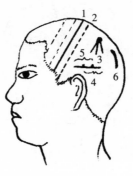

1. Motor region
2. Sensory region
3. Praxia region
4. Third speech region
5. Dizziness-hearing region
6. Second speech region

Fig. F–11. The lateral view of the stimulate regions

b. Indications:

    Apraxia (the patient cannot program dexterous and
    complex works, e.g., use a spoon or a fork for eat-
    ing or unbutton a button; the patient still has basic
    motor functions.

11. Balance region

   a.   Location: 3.5 cm. lateral to the apex of the exterior
occipital protuberance and stretching 4 cm. in length
(Fig. F–12).

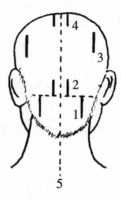

   1.   Balance region
   2.   Visual region
   3.   Second speech region
   4.   Foot motor-sensate region
   5.   Anterior–posterior middle line

Fig. F–12. The posterior view of stimulate regions

   b.   Indications

        Dysfunctions of the balance of the body due to dam-
aged cerebellum

12. Chest region

a. Location: Draw a horizontal line between the terminal point of the stomach region (6 cm. superior to the midpoint of the superior edge of the eyebrow) and anterior–posterior middle line; then extend 2 cm. up and 2 cm. down from the midpoint of the horizontal line. The chest region is 11 cm. in length (Fig. F–13).

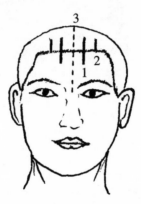

1. Chest region
2. Stomach region
3. Anterior–posterior middle line

Fig. F–13. The anterior view of the stimulate regions

b. Indications

Allergic asthma, chest pain; chest fullness; bronchial asthma; rheumatism of the heart (with clinical signs of restlessness, panting, edema and oliguria) and vetricular tachycardia

13. Stomach region

    a.   Location: 6 cm. superior to the middle of the superior edge of the eyebrow and extending up for 2 cm. (vertical to the pupil); Fig. F–14.

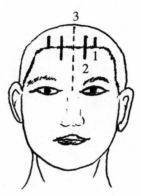

    1.   Stomach region
    2.   Chest region
    3.   Anterior–posterior middle line

Fig. F–14. The anterior view of stimulate regions

    b.   Indications

        Stomachache and stomach discomfort, especially from pain caused by acute or chronic gasteritis; also for ulceration of the stomach and duodenum (scalp acupuncture produces a remarkable effect).

14. Liver–gall bladder region

    a.   Location: The liver-gall bladder region is a line that extends from the end of the stomach region (Fig. F–15). It is 2 cm. in length and runs parallel to the anterior–posterior middle line.

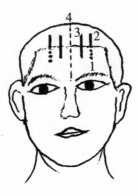

    1.   Liver–gall bladder area
    2.   Stomach region
    3.   Chest region
    4.   Anterior–posterior middle line

Fig. F–15. The anterior view of the stimulate regions

    b.   Indication:

        This region has a special use in the relief of pain in the right side of upper abdominal area due to liver and gall bladder disorders.

15. Intestinal region

a. Location: The intestinal region extends down from the end of the genital region (Fig. F–16 and 17). It is 2 cm. in length and runs parallel with the anterior–posterior middle line.

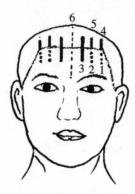

1. Intestinal region
2. Liver–gall bladder region
3. Chest region
4. Genital region
5. Stomach region
6. Anterior–posterior middle line

Fig. F–16. The anterior view of the stimulate region

b. Indications: Especially effective for the treatment of pain in the lower abdominal region.

16. Genital region

   a. Location: The genital region extends upward from the corner of the forehead. It is 2 cm. in length and runs parallel to the anterior–posterior middle line (Fig. F–17).

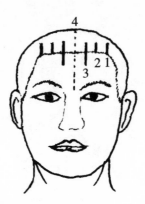

1.   Genital region
2.   Stomach region
3.   Chest region
4.   Anterior–posterior middle line

Fig. F–16. The anterior view of the stimulate region

   b. Indications:

    1) Functional uterine bleeding.

    2) In combination with the foot-sensate region for the treatment of polyuria due to acute cystitis.

    3) Thirst and polyuria due to diabetes.

    4) Seminal emission and impotence.

G. A General Introduction to Scalp Acupuncture Practice

1. The selection of needles

   a. Rapid perpendicular insertion: 0.5–1 cun in length; #26–28 in gauge (0.45–0.38 mm. in diameter)

   b. Slow oblique insertion 1.0–1.5 cun in length; #28–30 gauge (0.38–0.32 mm. in diameter)

   c. Acute syndromes: use a thicker needle

   d. Chronic syndromes: use a thinner needle

2. The position of the patient for needle insertion

   The position of the patient for needle insertion is not limited; the patient may be seated, standing, in a supine or a prone position.

   a. Whether the patient is standing, sitting or lying down for scalp acupuncture, the practitioner should stand and face the anterior, posterior or lateral views of the head of the patient. The practitioner should not be positioned in the direction of an inclined plane with the head of the patient.

   b. The patient does not have to sit or rest after needle insertion. Normal movement will facilitate the circulation of Qi and Blood and will enhance the therapeutic effect.

3. The principle of the selection of the stimulate region

   a. The selection of the stimulate region and the direction of the needle insertion have to be precise. The practitioner has to determine the length of the anterior–posterior middle line and the location of the eyebrow–occipital line. The stimulate regions (motor, sensory, or another region) can then be determined for needle insertion.

b.   Disorder in one side of the body: Insert needles in the
     stimulate region that is opposite to the side of the disorder.

c.   Disorder in both sides of the body: Insert needles in
     the stimulate regions of both sides of the body.

d.   The systemic disorders, for example, hypertension,
     asthma, urticaria, dermatitis, Mernier's syndrome and
     epilepsy, or those disorders whose symptomology is
     not limited to one particular side of the body: Insert
     needles on both sides of the stimulate regions.

e.   After needle insertion, the needle is moved to the
     proper depth in the direction of the stimulate region.

4.   Aseptic Procedure

Aseptic procedure for scalp acupuncture is the same as in
body or ear needle insertion. After the diagnosis and
selection of the stimulate region, the area is swabbed with
a 75% alcohol or a 2% iodine solution. The practitioner
must swab both hands with alcohol.

5.   The Method of Needle Insertion

The handle of the needle is held tightly by the thumb and
index finger. Insert the needle at the stimulate region at an
angle of 15–45° to the scalp and move the needle to the
layer of the epicranial aponeurosis. The length of the
needle body in the scalp has to cover the length of the
stimulate region. Manipulation of the needle is performed
after the entire length of the needle is inserted. If it is
necessary to insert the needle in the whole motor or
sensory region, the needles are inserted respectively at the
upper, middle and lower parts, one needle for each part.
The lift and thrust method of needle manipulation is not to
be applied.

Clinically, the flying needle insertion technique is used in
scalp acupuncture. This method can be used for perpendicular or oblique insertions and the patient feels little or

no pain sensation from the needle insertion. The procedure of flying needle insertion is as follows:

a.   Hold needle handle tightly with thumb and index finger.

b.   Rapidly insert the needle in the exact stimulate region, then,

   1)   Insert to a certain depth with one movement if it is a perpendicular needle insertion (Fig. G–1).

   2)   Move the needle along the direction of stimulate region for the whole length of the stimulate region (Fig. G–2). If the patient has too much pain from the needle movement or the needle is difficult to move, discontinue needle movement or change the needle direction and try again.

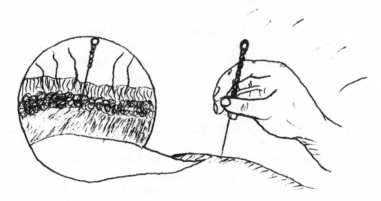

Fig. G–1. The Flying Needle Insertion in a Perpendicular Direction

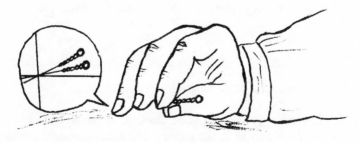

Fig. G–2. The Flying Needle Insertion with an Oblique Angle of Insertion

6. Manipulation of the Needle

    a. Lift and Thrust Method: This is usually used with an oblique angle of insertion. Move the needle up and down or move the scalp along the direction of the stimulate region to help the needle move up and down in the scalp.

    b. Pick Method: This is used for both perpendicular and oblique needle insertions. The needle is frequently picked in a small extent for a short period of time in each manipulation.

    c. Rotate Method: Slightly and slowly rotate the needle. This method can be combined with the lift and thrust method when strong stimulation is required to treat certain disorders.

    d. Electro-needle Stimulator: The frequency used is usually 200 c/m (cycles per minute) and the intensity is based on the tolerance of the patient. The time of stimulation is usually 20–30 minutes.

7. The Duration of Needle Retention

    The length of time that the needles are retained in place is based on several factors: the function of each stimulate region; the patient's body constitution; and the kind of disorder. In general, the needles are retained for longer periods of time in cases of pain and soreness, and for less time in cases of milder pain that is chronic in nature. Clinically, the duration of needle retention in scalp acupuncture therapeutics is twenty to thirty minutes.

8. The Intensity of Stimulation

    The intensity of stimulation can be determined by the needle sensation of the patient. The needle sensation in the stimulate region of the scalp is less distinct than the Qi

sensation at body points. Although most patients have no
prominent needle sensation from scalp acupuncture, the
effects of treatment are nonetheless remarkable. Clinically,
milder stimulation is given to elderly patients, weak
patients, and those patients with deficient syndromes and
who are prone to needle-fainting. The treatment of pain in
excessive syndromes requires more stimulation intensity.
Also, the intensity of stimulation from strong to mild has
to be changed as the patient recovers

9. Needle Sensation

The needle sensations produced by scalp acupuncture
therapeutics are experienced as heat, numbness and
twitching. Approximately eighty percent of patients
experience a mild heat sensation. Some patients have no
needle sensation, but still get a satisfactory therapeutic
effect. The needle sensation usually appears in the opposite
side of the limbs (the side of the disorder)while a few
patients have a needle sensation in the same side as the
needled stimulate region (the healthy side). The duration of
the needle sensation is from three to ten minutes but it can
extend for a few hours to two days.

10. Patient Reaction During or Following Scalp Acupuncture

The following describes the patient's reaction during or
after scalp acupuncture treatment:

a.   Uncontrolled motor reaction: The limbs of the side
     with the symptoms can be uncontrolled, lifting up,
     stretching or twitching during or after needling; the
     patient with paralysis in the lower limbs can have
     uncontrolled, muscle movement when standing or
     walking during or after treatment.

b.   Excessive sweating: This usually happens in the face
     or the palm of hand on the side of the disorder.

    c. Prominent recovery: About 10% of patients with paralysis have prominent recovery after the first treatment.

    d. Temporarily worse: A few patients could worsen after needle insertion, but after needle withdrawal, the patient will recover for a few minutes or hours.

11. The Interval of Needle Insertion and the Duration of Therapeutics

    a. The Interval of Needle Insertion

The interval of needle insertion is based on the conditions of different syndromes or disorders, and on the frequency of treatment whether once or twice a day, once every other day, or twice a week. Clinically, treatments are scheduled more closely for an initial period of time. As the patient begins to recover, the treatment interval is extended. For example, the treatment of hypertension, the interval of needle insertion is once every other day for several treatments, then once a month after the blood pressure has returned to a normal value and the symptoms of hypertension disappear.

    b. The Duration of Therapeutics

Clinically, each duration of therapeutics is three, six, ten, fifteen, or twenty treatments. If the patient has not recovered during the first duration of therapeutics, take a rest for one to two weeks, then give the second duration of therapeutics. The purpose of taking a rest between each duration of therapeutics is to avoid producing "needle resistance". When any single point has been used frequently for needle insertion, it will show a fatigue status and negatively effect the therapeutic effect. This is a common observation in clinical practice. The patient will have a remarkable response from the first or second treatment after which there is no improvement, even though the frequency of treatment is increased. Therefore, to avoid producing "needle resistance", both the interval of needle insertion and the duration of therapeutics are determined by the patient's tolerance of needle insertion and by the patient's condition as indicated by the symptoms and syndromes.

12. The Favorable Time of Needle Insertion

The timing of treatment has a great effect on the clinical results of scalp acupuncture therapeutics. In the case of a patient who has a disorder with a pronounced regularity of attack, treatment is given before the onset of the attack in order to prevent it from occurring and after an attack to relieve symptoms. These kinds of disorders include allergic asthma, bronchial asthma, chronic ulceration, epilepsy, hysteria, and periodic paralysis. The treatment of irregular menstruation and dysmenorrhea is best given one week before menstruation; the treatment of insomnia and nocturnal enuresis is best given one-half to one hour before bed. An understanding of the favorable time of needle insertion in scalp acupuncture therapeutics is an important element to grasp in order to enhance the clinical effect.

13. Withdrawal of the Needle

a.   Keep hair away from the needle with the fourth and fifth fingers.

b.   Hold the needle with the thumb and index finger (or thumb, index and middle fingers) and rapidly pull out the needle.

c.   To prevent bleeding at the site of puncture, it is necessary to press the puncture site gently with a sterilized dry cotton ball during and after withdrawal of the needle.

14. Precautions

    a.   The insertion site, including hair, needs to be clean before needle insertion.

    b.   Strict aseptic procedures are to be followed including swabbing with 75% alcohol or 2% iodine of the stimulate region, puncture site and hands of the practitioner.

    c.   The exact location of the stimulate region must be located.

    d.   Withdraw the needle with sterilized dry cotton ball to prevent bleeding at the puncture site.

    e.   Look at the patient's facial expression during needle manipulation.

    f.   In the treatment of CVA (cerebral vascular accident), the patient must be in a stable condition and show a consistent range of blood pressure.

    g.   If a paralysis patient presents with another syndrome, for example, edema, fever, acute inflammation, etc., treatment should address those syndromes first with body points; then begin treatment of paralysis with scalp acupuncture after those syndromes have been improved or cured.

    h.   To treat the paralysis patient, scalp acupuncture is given as well as physical exercise to enhance the therapeutic effect.

    i.   For the needle-fainting patient, withdraw the needle immediately and let the patient lay down. The patient will usually recover within a minute or two.

    j.   If the needle has bent or broken, the management is the same as in ordinary acupuncture.

Chapter X

Practical Ear Acupuncture

Therapeutics

CHAPTER X: PRACTICAL EAR ACUPUNCTURE
THERAPEUTICS

Ear acupuncture therapeutics is an important part of Chinese medical science. It is indicated in the first written record of Chinese medicine, the *Nei Jing* (1,200 - 4,000 B.C.), that the ear was not considered to be an individual organ, but was connected to all the organs of the body. The criteria and merits of ear needle therapy used in diagnosis and treatment were first presented in the *Chian Jin Fun (The Thousand Gold Recipes),* written by Sun Si-Mo of the early Tang dynasty in 652 A.D. Thus, the history of the ear acupuncture in Chinese medicine is well over 1,300 years old. In the past fifty years, the application of ear acupuncture to the diagnosis and treatment of various disorders has gained importance among acupuncturists.

At the present time, there are approximately two hundred points located on the ear. The names of the ear points reflect the phenomenology of the viscera in ancient Chinese medicine as well as the anatomic physiology of contemporary medicine. Ear acupuncture has many merits. These include a wide application in a variety of disorders, a rapid effect, convenience for the patient and a minimum of side-effects.

In order to strengthen the effect of ear acupuncture therapeutics, it is suggested that a practitioner consider using body needles and/or herbs in conjunction with the basic ear needle treatment for weight reduction, stop smoking, detoxification from drug abuse and mental depression. These are examples of some of the cases that have had a surprisingly satisfactory result from treatment using ear and body needles together.

The criteria and merits of ear acupuncture therapeutics have been presented. However, my colleagues and I have experienced some problems in the past eighteen years of practice. For example, ear needle therapy can only address the symptoms of certain diseases such as emphysema, epilepsy and chronic pain disorders. Also, the initial pain of insertion and the discomfort of the embedded needle may cause the patient to lose his confidence in this technique, especially during a long period of treatment. Further research is needed to improve this situation.

A. The Physiological Structure of the Auricle

The auricle consists of skin, fat, connective tissue, cartilage, nerves, blood vessels and lymphatic vessels. The lobule is the only part of the auricle that has no cartilage; it occupies one-fifth of the auricle. The nerve distribution on the auricle is very abundant, consisting of the trigeminal nerve, facial nerve, glosspharyneal nerve, vagus nerve, great auricular nerve, small occipital nerve and tempero-auricular nerve. Blood to the auricle is supplied by the posterior auricular artery, superficial temporal artery and superficial temporal veins. The lymphatic vessels of the auricle are very abundant and their distribution on the auricle is configured like a net. Their main function is to protect against infections in the auricle.

B. The Anatomical Structure of the Surface of the Auricle

The auricle is divided into seventeen parts in ear acupuncture as follows (Fig. B-1)

1. Helix: The prominent rim of the auricle.

2. Auricular tubercle: A small tubercle at the posterior upper part of the helix.

3. Scapha (Scaphoid fossa): The narrow crevice between the helix and the antihelix.

4. Tail of helix: On the border between the end of helix and lobule.

5. Lobule: The lower part of the auricle where is no cartilage.

6. Antihelix: A curved prominence opposite the helix.

7. Tragus: A small curved flap in front of the auricle.

8. Antitragus: A small tubercle opposite the tragus and inferior to the antihelix.

9. Intertragic notch: The depression between the tragus and the antitragus.

10. Orifice of the internal auditory meatus: Inside of the cavum conchae.

11. Cavum conchae: The concha inferior to the crux of the helix.

12. Crus of helix: The initial part of the helix.

13. Supratragic notch: The depression between the crus of the helix and the upper border of the tragus.

14. Cymba conchae: The concha superior to the crus of helix.

15. Inferior crus of antihelix: The inferior branch of the antihelix.

16. Superior crus of antihelix: The superior branch of the antihelix.

17. Triangular fossa: Between the superior and the inferior crus of the antihelix.

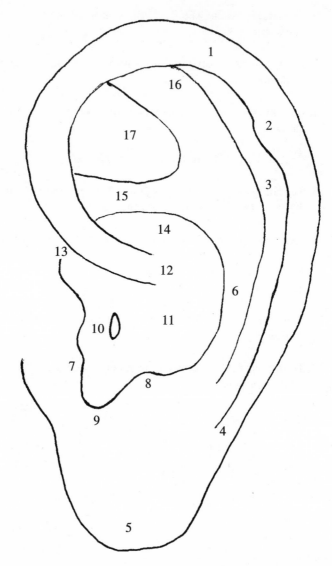

Fig. B–1. The Anatomical Structure of the Surface of the Auricle

C. The Relationship Between the Anatomical Structure of the Surface of the Auricle and Body Organs in Ear Acupuncture

The ear is not an individual organ but is connected to all the organs in the body. The points are distributed on the ear in the pattern of a fetus positioned upside down in the uterus with the head downward and the buttocks upward. This important concept underlies the point distribution on the auricle:

1. Lobule: Face region.

2. Antitragus: Head region.

3. Tragus: Nose and pharynx regions.

4. Around the cavum concha: Chest region including heart and lung.

5. Around the crus of helix: Digestive tract (mouth, esophagus, stomach, duodenum, small and large intestines, liver, gall bladder, pancreas, kidney and urinary bladder).

6. Cavum conchae: Liver, gall bladder, pancreas, kidney and urinary bladder.

7. Crus of helix: Diaphragm.

8. Triangular fossa: Genital organs

9. Inferior crus of antihelix: Buttocks region.

10. Superior crus of antihelix: Lower limbs.

11. Scapha: Upper limbs.

12. Antihelix: Spine.

D. The Location of Auricular Points (Fig. D-1)

Crus of the Helix

1. Center of ear: At the end of crus of helix.

2. Diaphragm: On the most part of crus of helix.

Helix

1. Lower part of the Rectum: At the anterior part of the helix on the same level are the Kidney point.

2. Urethra: On the helix level with the lower border of inferior crus of the antihelix.

3. Anus: In the middle between Urethra and lower part of the Rectum, on the same level as the Urinary Bladder point.

4. External Genital Organs: On the helix level with the upper border of the inferior crus of antihelix.

5. Ear Apex: At the tip of auricle when folded towards tragus.

6. Kanyan-1: At the helix above the level of the auricular tubercle.

7. Kanyan-2: At the helix on the lower margin of the auricular tubercle.

8. Helix-1,2,3,4,5,6: The region from the middle border of auricular tubercle (Helix-1) to the midpoint of lower border of lobule (Helix-6) is divided into five equal parts. The points marking the divisions are respectively Helix 2,3,4, and 5.

9. Tonsil-1,2,3,4: At the helix, a total of four points are respectively at the top, lateral and tall of helix, with an additional point on the lobule.

Scaphoid Fossa

1. Fingers: superior to the auricular tubercle in the scaphoid
    fossa.

2. Wrist: In the scaphoid fossa level with the lower border of
    the auricular tubercle.

3. Elbow: Between the Wrist and Shoulder points, level with
    the lower border of the inferior crus of the antihelix.

4. Shoulder: In the scaphoid fossa, level with supratragic
    notch.

5. Shoulder Joint: Between the Shoulder and Clavical points.

6. Clavicle: At the scaphoid fossa, level with the Neck point.

7. Nephritis Spot: At the infero-exterior part of the Clavicle
    point.

8. Appendix Spot: There are three spots in all: one located on
    the superior part of the fingers point; a second located on
    the superior of the Shoulder point; and a third point
    located on the inferior part of the Clavicle point.

9. Urticaria: In the scaphoid fossa at the mid-point between
    the fingers and wrist points.

Superior Crux of Antihelix

1. Toes: At the posterior upper corner of the superior crus of
    the antihelix.

2   Heel: at the antero-superior part of the superior crus of the
    antihelix.

3. Ankle Joint: At the inferior part between the Toes and Heel
    points.

4. Knee: At the origin of the superior crus of the antihelix level with the upper border of the inferior crus of the antihelix.

5   Coxa Joint: At the middle between the Toes, and Sacral Vertebra points.

6. Knee Joint: At the middle between Toes and Coxae Joint points.

Inferior Crus of Antihelix

1. Buttocks: On the origin of inferior crus of the antihelix.

2. Sympathetic Nerve: At the end of of the inferior crus of the antihelix.

3   Sciatic Nerve: The midpoint between the Buttocks and Sympathetic Nerve points.

Triangular Fossa

1. Shenmen: Inferior to 1/3 of the superior crus of the antihelix.

2. Uterus: At the midpoint of the inferior border of the helix.

3. Decreasing Blood Pressure Spot: At the border line between the superior curs of the antihelix and helix.

4. Asthma Spot: About 0.2 cm lateral to the Uterus point.

5. Hepatitis Spot: Midpoint between the Asthma Spot and Shenmen point.

Antihelix

1. Abdomen: Level with the lower border of the inferior crus of the antihelix.

2. Thorax: Level with the supratragic notch.

3. Neck: At the junction of the antihelix and antitragus.

4. Sacral Vertebrae: At the projection of the antihelix.

5. Cervical Vertebrae: At the projection of the antihelix.

6. Lumbar Vertebrae and 7. Thoracic vertebrae: Divide the area from the Sacral to Cervical Vertebrae into three equal parts; there are four points, the second and third of which are respectively the Lumbar and Thoracic Vertebrae points

Lobule

Note: From the end of the intertragic notch to end of the lobule draw three equal lines; then, draw two vertical lines to divide the lobule into nine areas (sections).

1. Eye-1, Eye-2: On both sides of the intertragic notch, the anterior point being Eye-1 and the posterior being Eye-2.

2. Toothache-1: At the postero-inferior corner of the first section of the lobule.

3. Toothache-2: In the center of the fourth section of the lobule.

4. Lower Jaw: At the antero-superior part of the second section.

5. Upper Jaw: at the postero inferior part of the second section.

6. Maxilla: at the midpoint of the third section.

7. Mandible: at the midpoint of the superior line of the third section.

8. Tongue: in the center of section two.

9. Eye: at the midpoint of section five.

10. Internal ear: at the midpoint of section six.

11. Tonsils: at the midpoint of section eight.

12. Special Area of Tumor: this area is from Helix-4 to Helix-6 points.

Tragus

1. External Nose: in the center of the lateral side of the tragus.

2. Pharynx and Larynx: in the upper half of the medial aspect of the tragus.

3. Internal Nose: in the medial and inferior aspect of the tragus.

4. Apex of Tragus: at the upper tubercle on the border of the tragus.

5. Adrenal Gland: at the lower tubercle on the border of the tragus.

6. Thirst Spot: At the midpoint between the Apex of tragus and the External Nose points.

7. Hungry Spot: At the midpoint between the Adrenal Gland and the External Nose points.

Intertragic Notch

Internal Secretions: at the bottom part of the intertragic notch toward the tragus.

Antitragus

1. Asthma (pinchung): at the middle of the brim of the antitragus.

2. Subcortex: on the interior wall of the antitragus.

3. Brain Stem: at the junction of the antitragus and antihelix; this point is toward the antihelix, and the neck point is toward the scaphoid fossa.

4. Brain Spot: At the midpoint between the Asthma (Pinchung) and the Brain Stem points.

5. Ovary: At the lower part of the interior wall of the antitragus.

6. Forehead: At the antero-inferior corner of the lateral aspect of the antitragus.

7. Occiput: At the postero-superior corner of the lateral aspect of the antitragus.

8. Taiyang: At the midpoint between the Forehead and Occiput points.

Periphery of the Crus of Helix

1. Stomach: At the area where the crus of helix terminates.

2. Duodenun: At the posterior third of the superior aspect of the crus of helix.

3. Small Intestine: At the middle third of the superior aspect of the crus of helix.

4. Large Intestine: At the anterior third of superior aspect of the crus of helix.

5. Appendix: At the midpoint between the Large Intestine and Small Intestine points.

6. Mouth: Close to the posterior wall of the orifice of the external auditory meatus.

7. Esophagus: At the upper part of the cavum conchae just below the disappearance of the crus of helix.

8. Cardiac Orifice: Behind the esophagus point,at the upper part of the cavum conchae just below the crus of helix.

Cavum Conchae

1. Heart: In the center of the cavum conchae (the deepest depression of the cavum conchae).

2. Lung Area: Around the heart point.

3. Trachea: Between the mouth and heart points.

4. Sanjiao: Forming a triangle with the Mouth and Heart points.

5. Spleen: Inferior to Liver point, close to the border of the antihelix.

6. Hepatic Cirrhosis: At the lateral side between the lower part of the Hepatomegalia and Stomach points just below the disappearance of the crus of helix.

7. Hepatitis Area: Between the stomach and spleen points and slightly inferior.

Cymba Conchae

1. Prostate: Below the Sympathetic Nerve point.

2. Bladder: On the lower border of the inferior crus of the antihelix directly above the Large Intestine point.

3. Kidney: On the lower border of the Inferior crus of the antihelix directly above the Small Intestine point.

4. Pancreas and Gall Bladder: Between the Liver and Kidney points.

5. Liver: Posterior to the stomach and duodenum points; these three points form a triangle.

6. Ascites Spot: Among the Kidney, Pancreas and Gall Bladder, and Small Intestine Points.

Back of the Auricle

1. Upper Back: On the protuberance of cartilage on the upper part of the back of the auricle.

2. Lower Back: On the protuberance of cartilage at the lower part of the back of the auricle.

3. Middle Back: At the midpoint of the line connecting the two points of the upper and lower back of the auricle.

4. Groove for Decreasing Blood Pressure: In the groove between the lateral border of the protuberance of the cartilage and helix.

5. Root of the Auricular Vagus Nerve: At the junction of the back of the auricle and mastoid level with the crus of helix.

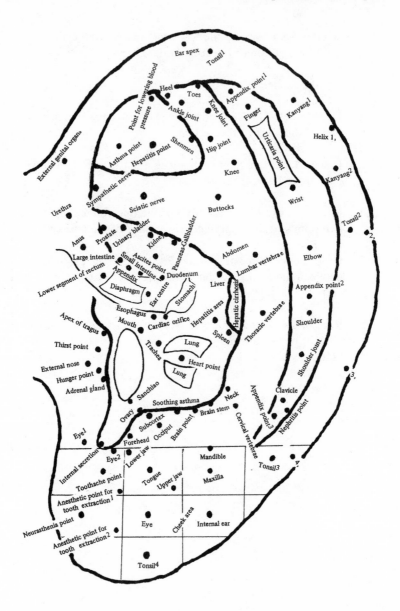

Fig. D–1. The Location of Auricular Points

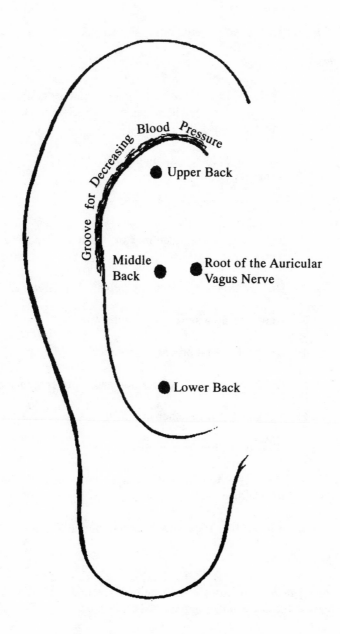

Fig. D–2. The Back of the Auricle

E. The Indications of the Auricular Points

Crus of the Helix

1. Center of Ear: Disorders of the circulatory system.
    This functions much the same as the triple warmer
    point (Sanjiao).

2. Diaphragm: Hiccup, jaundice and skin and blood
    disorders.

Helix

1. Lower Part of the Rectum: Constipation, diarrhea and
    hemorrhoid.

2. Urethra: Retention of urine, polyuria and urethritis.

3. Anus: Burning sensation of anus.

4. External genital organs: Impotence

5. Ear Apex: Fever, hypertension and acute conjunctivitis

6. Kanyan-1: Chronic hepatitis.

7. Kanyan-2:Chronic hepatitis

8. Helix 1-6: Acute tonsillitis, hypertension and various
    febrile disorders.

9. Tonsils 1-4: Tonsillitis and pharyngolaryngitis.

Scaphoid Fossa

The following points are indicated for treatment of pain disorders at the corresponding part of the body.

1. Fingers

2. Wrist

3. Elbow

4. Shoulder

5. Shoulder joint

6. Clavicle

7. Nephritis Spot: Nephritis

8. Appendix Spot : Appendicitis

9. Urticaria Area: Urticaria

Superior Crus of the Antihelix

The following points address pain and other disorders at the corresponding part of the body.

1. Toes

2. Heel

3. Ankle joint

4. Knee

5. Coxa joint

6. Knee joint

Inferior Crus of Antihelix

1. Buttock: Pain and disorders at the corresponding part of the body.

2. Sympathetic Nerve: Excessive sweating, stomach spasm and other disorders of the digestive and circulatory system.

3. Sciatic Nerve: Sciatica

Triangular Fossa

1. Shenmen: Mental disorders, dry cough, epilepsy, insomnia, inflammatory disorders, functions in sedation, harmonizes with liver.

2. Uterus: Irregular menstruation, leukorrhea, dysmenorrhea, and impotence.

3. Decreasing Blood Pressure Spot: Hypertension

4. Asthma Spot: Asthma, chronic cough and shortness of breath.

5. Hepatitis Spot: Acute and chronic hepatitis.

Antihelix

1. Abdomen: Abdominal distention, pain and dysmenorrhea

2. Thorax: Chest fullness or pain and intercostal neuralgia

3. Neck: Neck stiffness and neck pain.

4. Sacral Vertebrae: Pain in the buttock and sacral vertebrae.

5. Cervical Vertebrae: Neck pain and pain in the cervical vertebrae.

6. Lumbar Vertebrae: Pain in the lower back and lumbar vertebrae

7. Thoracic Vertebrae: Pain in the upper and middle parts of the back and pain in thoracic vertebrae.

Lobule

1. Eye-1 and Eye-2: Glaucoma and myopia.

2. Toothache-1: Toothache and other tooth disorders.

3. Toothache-2: Toothache and other tooth disorders.

The following five points are indicated for the treatment of pain or disorders at the corresponding part of the body:

1. Lower Jaw

2. Upper Jaw

3. Maxilla

4. Mandible

5. Tongue

6. Eye: Eye disorders

7. Internal Ear: Impaired heariang and tinnitus

8. Tosils: Tonsilitis

9. Special Area of Tumor

10. Internal Ear: Impaired heariang and tinnitus

11. Tonsils: Tonsilitis

12. Special area of tumor: Various tumors

Tragus

1. External Nose: Sinusitis

2. Pharynx and larynx: pharyngitis, laryngitis and tonsilitis.

3. Internal Nose: Sinusitis

4. Apex of the Tragus: Toothache

5. Adrenal Gland: Hypotension, allergic disorders, inflammatory disease, shock, fever, skin disease, various chronic disorders, cough, asthma and poison.

6. Thirsty: Diabetes and weight loss

7. Hungry spot: diabetes and weight loss

Intertragic Notch

Internal Secretion: Hematologic disease, endocrine disturbances, antiallergic and antirheumatic disease and skin disease.

Antitragus

1. Asthma (Pinching): Asthma, bronchitis and mumps

2. Subcortex: Inflammatory disease, various pains, insomnia, dream-disturbed sleep and mental illness.

3. Brain stem: Polyhydrosis, shock, excessive sweating, enuresis and hemiplegia.

4. Brain spot: Same as brain stem

5. Ovary: irregular menstruation.

6. Forehead: Headache, dizziness, insomnia, neurasthenia and sinusitis.

7. Occiput: Headache, neck stiffness and cough.

8. Taiyang: Migraine headache and enuresis

Periphery of the Crus of Helix

1. Stomach: Vomiting, dyspepsia and gastralgia.

2. Duoenum: ulceration of duoenum.

3. Small Intestine: Indigestion, abdominal distention and dyspepsia.

4. Large Intestine: Diarrhea, indigestion and enteritis.

5. Appendix: Appendicitis.

6. Mouth: Facial paralysis

7 Esophagus: Esophagitis.

8. Cardiac Orifice: Cardiac disorders, palpitation, chest pain, night sweating, insomnia and excessive dreaming.

Cavum Conchae

1. Heart: Anxiety, regulates blood circulation, tranquilizes mind, and various heart diseases.

2. Lung Area: Asthma, asthma, quit smoking, skin disease, shortness of breath, regulates Qi and various respiratory diseases.

3. Trachea: cough.

4. Sanjiao: Pain in the chest or abdomen, anemia, hepatitis, indigestion, edema and OBS disorders.

5. Spleen: Indigestion, gastritis, uterine bleeding, anemia, muscular atrophy or weakness, chronic diarrhea, strengthens Qi.

6. Hepatic Cirrhosis: Chronic hepatitis and cirrhosis.

7. Hepatitis Area: Hepatitis.

Cymba Conchae

1. Prostate: Prostatitis.

2. Urinary Bladder: Retention of urine; enuresis.

3. Kidney: Impaired hearing, lower back pain, nephritis, pyelitis, cystitis, strengthens Yang Qi

4. Pancreas and Gall Bladder: Pancreatitis, dyspepsia, gall stone, tinnitus and migraine headache.

5. Liver: Acute and chronic hepatitis, jaundice, weak eyesight, functions in control muscles and regulates blood.

6. Ascites Spot: Ascites

Back of the Auricle:

1. Upper back: Upper back pain and itching.

2. Lower back: Lower back pain and itching.

3. Middle back: Middle back pain and itching.

4. Groove for Decreasing Blood Pressure: Hypertension.

5. Root of Auricular Vagus Nerve: Stomachache, asthma and headache.

F. Inspection of the Ear for Diagnosis

A visual inspection of the auricle provides diagnostic information that enables the practitioner to further assess the pathological condition. Needling at the exact pathological reaction spot produces the best results.

1. Acute inflammatory disease: Red papules (not painful), cappillaried, or painful red pimples.

2. Recent acute inflammatory disease: Glossy surface with redness.

3. Chronic inflammatory disease: Non-glossy surface with redness.

4. Chronic disease of the organs: White spot of furfur, depression, proturbance and white papule in corresponding organ.

5. Dermal disease or disease of the compensatory and absorbent dysfunction: Furfuranceous desquamation (difficult to eradicate).

6. All kinds of postoperations: White shallow scar, semicircular scale or dark gray scar in corresponding region of operation.

7. Tumor: Dark gray spot and furfur or protuberant nodule.

G. Auricular Tender Spots:

There are many different kinds of instruments to use to inspect the ear for tender spots from the simple detector, such as the head of a needle (round shape) to the complex detector such as the electric machine. (See Fig. G-1)

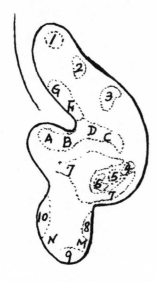 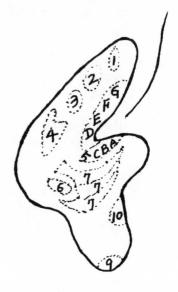

Left Ear Cavity (Enlarge)   RightEar Cavity (Enlarge)

1. Urinary bladder   1. Urinary bladder
2. Kidney   2. Kidney
3. Pancreas and Gall Bladder   3. Pancreas and Gall Bladder
4. Liver   4. Liver
5. Spleen   5. Digestive Tract:
6. Heart   A. Esphagus
7. Lung   B. Cardiac Orifice
8. Subcortex   C. Stomach
9. Internal secretion   D. Duodenum
10. Internal nose   E. Small Intestine
11. Digestive tract   F. Appendix
    A. Esophagus   G .Large Intestine
    B. Cardiac orifice   6. Heart
    C. Stomach   7. Lung
    D. Duodenum   8. Subcortext
    E. Small Intestine   9. Internal secretion
    F. Appendix   10. Internal Nose
    G. Large Intestine
M. Ovary
N. Adrenal Gland

Fig. G–1. The Auricular Tender Spots

H. The Twelve Sensitive Points

There are twelve specific points known as "sensitive points" that are widely used in clinical practice with remarkable results in treating many different kinds of disorders.

Fig. H-1 shows the location of the twelve sensitivie points in the auricle:

Auricular apex point

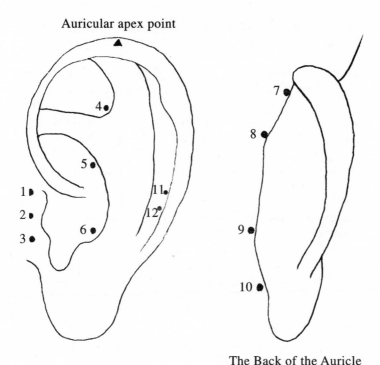

The Back of the Auricle

Fig. H–1. The Twelve Sensitive Points in the Auricle

1. Sensitive-1 point: On the superior corner of the lateral aspect of tragus, close to the supratragic notch.

2. Sensitive-2 point: On the middle part of the lateral aspect of tragus.

3. Sensitive-3 point: On the inferior corner of the lateral aspect of tragus, close to the junction of tragus and intertragic notch.

4. Sensitive-4 point: On the postero-inferior part of triangular fossa, vertical to the auricular apex point.

5. Sensitive-5 point: in the symba conchae, directly below the fourth point, vertical to the auricular apex point.

6. Sensitive-6 point: On the postero-inferior part of cavum conchae.

7. Sensitive-7 point: On the back of auricle, the point is in the upper part of the junction of the back of auricle and mastoid.

8. Sensitive-8 point: On the junction of the back of auricle and mastoid, one cun (about 2.5 cm) away from the 7th point.

9. Sensitive-9 point: On the junction of the back of auricle and mastoid, 1.3 cun (about 2.8 cm) away from the 8th point.

10. Sensitive-10 point: In the back of lobule, just the end of the lower part of cartilage.

11. Sensitive-11 point: In the interior aspect of helix, level with the supratragic notch.

12. Sensitive-12 point: In the interior aspect of helix, level with the middle of the brim of tragus.

The Functions of the Twelve Sensitive Points

Diseases	Prescriptions
Arthritis	Sensitive- 1, 4, 5, 6, 7, 8, 9, 10
Circulatory disease	Sensitive- 1, 2, 6. 7, 8, 9
Digestive disease	Sensitive- 5, 6, 7, 8, 9, 10, 11, 12
Facial spasm	Sensitive- 1, 2, 3, 5, 6
Myasthenia	Sensitive- 1, 4, 5, 6, 7, 9, 10
Nervous dysfunction	Sensitive- 3, 5, 6, 7, 9, 10
Neurasthenia	Sensitive- 1, 3, 5, 7, 8, 9, 10
Rheumatoid arthritis	Sensitive- 6, 7, 9, 10, 11, 12
Rheumatic pain	Sensitive- 1, 2, 3, 4, 5, 6, 7, 9
Sciatica	Sensitive- 1, 6, 7

I.   General Introduction To Ear Acupuncture Practice

1.   The Principle of Selection of Ear points

   a.   Based on the location of disease: most ear points, or
        reaction spots, correspond to certain parts of the body,
        e.g. the wrist point, the liver point, the lung area, the
        kidney, etc. Points are selected according to the
        corresponding part of the body in which the disease is
        located.

   b.   Based on the theory of Chinese medical science: one
        of the basic principles of Chinese medicine is known
        as the external-internal relationship. The Lung, for
        example, has an external-internal relationship with the

Large Intestine; the Spleen is related to the Stomach, the Heart with the Small Intestine, the Kidney with the Urinary Bladder; and the Liver with the Gall Baldeder. Also, each organ is associated with a sensory ogran. The Lung opens to the nose; the Spleen opens to the mouth; the Heart opens to the tongue; the Kidney opens to the ear; and the Liver opens to the eyes. Therefore, the Lung point is chosen for treating disorders of the nose, the Spleen point for disorders of the mouth; the Heart point for disorders of the tongue; the Kidney point for disorders of the ear and the Liver point for disorders of the eye.

c. Based on the main physiological function of the internal organs: ear points are selected according to which organ is showing dysfunction.

   1) Lung: Dominating Qi and controlling respiration; regulating water passage and deminating the skin and hair.

   2) Spleen: Governing transportation and transformation; controlling blood and dominating the muscles.

   3) Heart: Controlling blood and vessels and housing the mind.

   4) Kidney: Storing essence and dominating reproduction, growth and development; producing marrow and dominating the bones; and dominating water metabolism.

   5) Liver: Storing blood, maintaining potency for the flow of Qi and controlling tendons.

d. Based on clinical experience: a practitioner's clinical experience provides valuable information for the use of ear acupuncture. Some commonly sued points are: Shenmen for emotional conditions and sedation; the Heart point for a peaceful spirit and a tranquil mind; the Lung area for smoking cessation; the thirsty and hungry spots for weight loss; and the Adrenal Gland for detoxification from substance abuse (drugs and alcohol).

2. Aseptic Procedure: Asepic procedures for ear acupuncture are the same as for any other needle insetion. Ear points are swabbed with 75% alcohol or 2% iodine.

3. The Method of Needle Insertion:

    a. The needles perpendicularly at points located on the symba conchae, cavum conchae and crus of helix. Insert needles obliquely (30 - 75%) at points located on all other parts of the ear.

    b. Speed of insertion: Rapidly insert the needle at the exact point location. This technique reduces the pain sensation from the needle insertion and enhances the therapeutic effect.

    c. Depth of insertion: The needle has to be inserted to the cartilage or should penetrate the cartilage, but not penetrate the other side of the skin. The deeper the insertion, the better the result.

4. The Order of Needle Insertion

    The acupuncture needles are inserted from the upper to the lower part of the ear and from the right to the left side of the ear (if the practitioner is right-handed). The needle should not touch each other when they are in place.

5. Manipulation of the Needle

    There is usually no mainpulation of ear nedles after insertion. Ear needles are not placed deep enough for twisting or lifting and thrusting manipulation. Electro-acupuncture and moxibustion are applicable instead of hand manipulation and are especially effective in the treatment of smoking cessation and substance abuse.

6. Needle Sensation: Ear acupuncture produces a sensation of warmth, soreness and distention. The greater the needle sensation, the better the clinical result.

7. Manipulation Methods for Tonification and Dispersion

   a. Tonification: Actively and frequently rub both ears until the patient has a feeling of warmth in the ear. The purpose of rubbing both ears before needle insertion is to warm the meridians in the body since ear points correspond to all the meridians of the body. After rubbing, insert the ear needles in both ears.

   b. Dispersion:

      1) Insert ear needles in one ear for thirty minutes or longer (for this example the needles are inserted in the right ear).

      2) Actively and frequently rub the ear (left ear) that does not have the needles for 1-3 minutes at intervals of ten minutes.

      3) Withdraw the needles from the right ear and insert clean needle in other ear (left ear) for 20 minutes or longer.

      4) Actively and frequently rub the ear (right ear) that does not have the needles (the purpose of rubbing the ear that does ot have the needles is to reinforce a needle sensation in the other ear that stimulates the meridians for dispersion.

8. The Interval of Needle Insertion and Duration of Therapeutics

   The frequency of treatment with ear acupuncture is determined by the nature of different syndromes or disorders. Treatment may be once a day, once every other day, or once every few days. Clinically, treatment is given more frequently at the beginning of a new case or in special cases such as stop smoking and detoxification. Extend the internal of treatment as the patient recovers in order to avoid the overuse of ear points. This is known as "point fatigue" or "needle resistance" and it negatively effects the therapeutic effect.

Each course of ear acupuncture treatments consists of two, six, eight or ten treatments given once every other day or every few days depending on the syndrome of disorder. If a patient still does not recover or cure from first duration of therapeutics, take rest for 1-2 weeks then give the second duration of therapeutics for avoid needle resistance and enhance therapeutics effect.

9. Withdrawal of Needle

   a.   Holding the needle with the thumb and index finger, pull the needle out rapidly.

   b.   To prevent bleeding at the site of puncture, it is necessary to press the puncture site with a sterilized dry cotton ball after withdrawal of the needle.

10. Contraindications:

   a.   In the treatment of pregnant women from the fifth to ninth months of pregnancy, no needling or imbedding needle in the points of uterus, ovary, internal secretion and abdomen to avoid miscarriage.

   b.   An extremely weakened condition or severe anemia.

   c.   Severe infections in the ear.

   d.   The patient who faints easily from needles.

   e.   No imbedding needle in an excessivly nervous patient.

   f.   Insert needles in the sympathetic, adrenal gland and internal secretion points for treating the patient who has headache, vertigo, vomiting or nausea during or after ear needling.

11. Imbedding Ear Needle Therapeutics

    a. Types of needles

        1) Thumbtack type: this needle is 0.2-0.6 cm long with a head like a thumbtack.

        2) Staple type: this needle is 0.3-0.4 cm long. It is suitable for imbedding in an ear spot or area, for example, thirsty or hungry spots, the lung area, the stomach area, urticaria, or the special tumor area.

        3) Grain-like type: this needle is about one-half to one cm. long with a head like a grain of wheat. This needle and the thumbtack needle are the most commonly used ear needles.

    b. Indications

    Chronic diseases of the internal organs; persistant pain disorders; epilepsy; asthma; arthritis; hysteria; special cases such as weight loss, smoking cessation, alcoholism, drug abuse and detoxification.

    c. The method of imbedding needles

        1) Strict antisepsis must be followed to avoid infection.

        2) Confirm the exact point location.

        3) Clip the needle with a forceps and insert it at the point.

        4) Cover the needle with a 75% alcohol cotton ball, press lightly and rub the top of the cotton ball to stimulate the imbedded needle for thirty seconds to one minute.

     5)   Remove the cotton ball.

     6)   Ask the patient to keep the ear dry while the needle is imbedded.

d. Retention of imbedding needle

The length of time during which ear needles are imbedded is determined by the kind of disease, the season, the course of treatment, and the tolerance to the imbedding needle of each patient.

The duration of implantation is from one to seven days. This period of time is shorter in the summer and in acute conditions; it is longer in the autumn and winter season, and in chronic conditions or specific cases, for example, drug abuse, detoxification, smoking cessation, and weight loss.

e. Removal of the needle

     1) Pinch one corner of the tape with a forceps and pull the whole tape from the surface of the ear.

     2) Pinch the needle head with a forceps and remove the needle. Clean the needle hole with a 75% alcohol cotton ball

J.   Ear and Body Points Used in the Treatment of Common Disease

In order to strengthen the therapeutic effect, it is suggested that
body points be used in conjunction with ear points.

<u>The Diseases of the Digestive System</u>

    1.   Abdominal distention

        Ear points: stomach, small intestines, sanjiao,
                       sympathetic nerve

        Body points: St 36, CV 12, St 25

    2.   Alcoholism

        Ear Points: forehead, subcortex, shenmen, occiput

        Body points: GV 26, GV 25

    3.   Diarrhea

        Ear points: small intestine, large intestine, spleen,
                       sympathetic nerve

        Body points: St36, St25, St 44, CV12

    4.   Enteritis

        Ear points: small intestine, large intestine,
                       sympathetic nerve

        Body points: St 36, St 25, LI 11, Pc 6

    5.   Gastritis

        Ear points: stomach, spleen, sympathetic nerve, shenmen

        Body points: St 36, CV 12, Liv 13

6. Stomachache

   Ear Points: stomach, shenmen

   Body points: St 34, Pc 6

7. Indigestion

   Ear point: small intestine, stomach, spleen, pancrease
                  and gall bladder

   Body points: St36, CV12, CV4, Pc6, St25

8. Nausea and Vomiting

   Ear points: stomach, shenman, sympathetic nerve,
                  occiput

   Body points: St36, Pc6, Sp4, St25

9. Constipation

   Ear points: large intestine, lower part of rectum,
                  subcortex

   Body points: TW 6, GB 34, Sp 15

10. Chronic Cholcystitis

    Ear Points: pancreas and gall bladder, liver, sympathetic
                   nerve, lung

11. Pancreatitis

    Ear points: pancreas, internal secretion, sympathetic
                   nerve, shenman

The Diseases of the Respiratory System

1. Asthma

    Ear points: lung, sympathetic nerve, shenmen,
                  pingchuan, kidney

    Body points: CV 17, St 40, Lu 9, UB 13, UB 23

2. Bronchitis

    Ear points: lung, pingchuan, adrenal gland

    Body points: GV 22, St 40, CV 17, GV 12

3. Chest pain

    Ear points: chest, shenmen, lung, heart, sympathetic
                  nerve

    Body points: Pc 6, TW 6, CV 6, TW 8

4. Common cold:

    Ear points: forehead, adrenal gland, lung

    Body points: UB 12, Lu 7, L.I. 20, GV 16, GB 20, St 36

5. Cough

    Ear Points: pingchung, adrenal gland, lung, shenmen

    Body points: CV 22, Pc 6, CV 17, UB 13, St 40

6. Whooping cough

    Ear points: bronchi, adrenal gland, pingchuan, lung,
                  sympathetic nerve

    Body Points: UB 13, Lu 1, Ki 6, Lu 6, Lu 7, CV 17

<u>The Disease of the Circulatory System</u>

1. Hypertension

   Ear points: depressing blood pressure groove,
                 shenmen, sympathetic nerve, heart

   Body points: L.I. 11, Liv 3, GB 20, St 36, Sp 6

2. Hypotension

   Ear points: heart, sympathetic nerve, adrenal gland,
                 subcortex

   Body points: GV 25, GV 26, Liv 3, Pc 6, TW 6

3. Hypoferric Anemia

   Ear points: spleen, liver, internal secretion, stomach,
                 small intestine

   Body Points: L.I. 4, GB 20, Pc 6, St 36, L.I. 11

4. Myocarditis

   Ear Points: heart, sympathetic nerve, small intestine,
                 spleen

5. Pulseless disease

   Ear points: sympathetic nerve, kidney, heart, adrenal
                 gland, liver, subcortex

6. Premature contraction

   Ear Points: heart, sympathetic nerve, small intestine,
                 subcortex, shenmen

   Body points: Ht 7, Pc 6

7. Tachycardia

    Ear points: heart, sympathetic nerve, shenman,
                  small intestine, subcortex

    Body Points: Ht 7, Pc 6, CV 17, UB 22, CV 14, UB 15

The Disease of the Nervous System

1. Headache

    Ear points: Occiput, Forehead, Shenman, Subcortex

    Body points

    1) Occipital headache: UB 10, UB 65, S.I. 3

    2) Frontal headache: St 8, Yintang, St 44, L.I. 4,
            Sp 4

    3) Migraine headache: Taiyang, GB 8, GB 41, GB 31

    4) Parietal headache: GV 20, S.I. 3, Liv 3

2. Dizziness

    Ear points: occiput, forehead, shenmen, subcortex,
                  heart, adrenal gland, internal secretion

    Body points: GB 20, Pc 6, Liv 3, GB 20, Yintang,
                 Taiyang

3. Dreams

    Ear points: shenmen, occiput, heart, kidney, sanjiao

4. Facial paralysis

    Ear Points: cheek, adrenal gland, subcortex, sanjiao

    Body points: TW 17, St 6, St 7, S.I. 18

5. Facial Spasm

   Ear Points: cheek, shenmen, subcortex

   Body points: Taiyang, St 6, St 7, L.I. 4

6. Epilepsy

   Ear points: shenmen, occiput, subcortex,
                 sympathetic nerve, heart, stomach

   Body points: St 36, Pc 6, GB 30, Liv 3, L.I. 4

7. Hysteria

   Ear points: shenmen, occiput, heart, stomach

   Body points: GV 26, Ht 7, Pc 6, GB 34

8. Insomnia

   Ear points: shenmen, kidney, occiput, heart,
                 subcortex

   Body points: Ht 7, Sp 6, St 36

9. Intercostal neuralgia

   Ear points: shenmen, thorax, lung

   Body points: TW6, GB34, TW8

10. Sciatica

    Ear Points: sciatic nerve, kidney, shenmen

    Body points: GB30, GB34, GB31, UB60, UB54

11. Neurasthenia

    Ear points: shenman, subcortex, heart, kidney, stomach

    Body points: Ht7, GB20, St36, Sp6, CV4

12. Polyhydrosis (excessive sweating in the palms of hands or soles of feet)

    Ear points: adrenal gland, sympathetic nerve, internal secretion, lung, kidney, shenmen, occiput

    Body points: Pc6, TW5, L.I.4, S.I.3

13. Shock

    Ear points: adrenal gland, occiput, heart, brain stem, subcortex

    Body points: L.I.4, GV26, GB20, Ki1, Ht8

14. Neck pain or stiffness

    Ear points: shenmen, neck, neck vertebra

    Body points: GB34, GB20, GB39, Liv1, Lu7

15. Trigeminal Neuralgia

    Ear points: cheek, shenmen, occiput, maxilla, mandible

    Body points: St7, L.I.20, St6, L.I.11, L.I.4

16. CVA (Cerebral vascular accident)

    Ear points: shenmen, subcortex, brain stem, ear apex

    Body points: GV20, GB20, Ki1, Liv3, L.I.4

17. Hemiplegia

    Ear points: Subcortex, sympathetic nerve, shenmen, adrenal gland

    Body points: L.I. 4, Ht3, Pc7, L.I.15, GB34, GV20, Sp6

The Diseases of Obstetrics and Gynecology

1. Dysmenorrhea

    Ear Points: uterus, internal secretion, sympathetic nerve, ovary

    Body Points: Sp6, Sp10, CV4, CV6, Sp4, St36

2. Irregular menstruation

    Ear Points: uterus, internal secretion, ovary, kidney

    Body points: CV4, Sp6, St36

3. Amenorrhea

    Ear points: uterus, internal secretion, ovary,kidney

    Body points: Sp6, CV4, St36, Sp10

4. Leukorrhea

    Ear points: uterus, internal secretion, ovary

    Body points: Sp6, CV6, St29

The Disease of the Urinary and Generative Systems

1. Cystitis

    Ear points: urinary bladder, kidney, occiput, adrenal
                    gland, sympathetic nerve

    Body points: UB23, UB26, UB28, CV3, Sp6, Sp9

2. Impotence

    Ear points: internal secretion, external genital organs,
                    uterus, kidney

    Body points: CV4, Sp6, CV2, CV3

3. Enuresis

    Ear points: urinary bladder, brain stem, occiput, kidney

    Body points: CV3, Sp6, UB23, St36

4. Prostatitis

    Ear points: prostate, urinary bladder, internal secretion,
                    adrenal gland, sympathetic nerve, kidney

    Body points: CV4, Liv3, Sp9, UB54

The Diseases of the Endocrine System

1. Diabetes

    Ear Points: thirsty, hungry, gall bladder and pancreas,
                    internal secretion, kidney

    Body points: Sp6, Sp9, St36, UB23

2. Hyperthyroidism

   Ear points: internal secretion, sympathetic nerve,
                 shenmen, kidney

   Body points: Sp3, L.I.5, TW17

Miscellaneous

1. Weight loss

   Imbedding needles in Sympathetic nerve, Pancreas and
   Gall Bladder, Adrenal Gland, Stomach, Thirsty ad Hungry
   spots, once a week in each duration of treatment.

2. Stop smoking

   Imbedding needles in Occiput, Lung, Shenmen, Sympathetic Nerve, and Kidney, once a week in each duration of
   treatment. Body points are GB20, CV4, Pc6, GB31, Ki3,
   and Liv3 for mental complications from quitting smoking;
   treat once a week in each duration of treatment to enhance
   the therapeutic effect.

3. Drug Abuse and Detoxification

   Ear points: sympathetic nerve, adrenal gland, sanjiao,
                 liver, subcortex, shenman, internal
                 secretion, kidney

   Body points: Liv 3, Ki 3, Sp 6, Sp 10, GB 31, CV 4, L.I. 4,
                Liv 13, UB 15, UB 23

   The needling in the above three cases are imbedding
   needle: needle groups of points alternatively once a week
   for several treatments. The body points are needled once a
   week in weight loss and in stop smoking treatments, and
   once every other day or twice a week in drug abuse and
   detox treatments.

K. The Pathways of the Meridians in the Auricle
(Fig. K-1, 2, 3, 4, 5, 6)

There are six Yang meridians that pass through the auricle from the body. More clinical research is needed to confirm the locations of these pathways. Although six Yin meridians do not directly pass through the auricle, they are connected to the Yang meridians and go indirectly to the auricle. The extra-meridians, such as the Yangchiao Mo, are respectively connected with the twelve regular meridians and go into the back of the auricle.

The regular meridians as well as the extra meridians directly or indirectly connect to the auricle from distributing over the body; they serve as a pathway of energy and as a bridge between the internal organs and the surface of the body.

Pathological changes in the internal organs will appear as pathological reaction spots in the corresponding part of the surface of the body. The ear is not an individual organ but is connected with the organs in the body as indicated in the *Nei Jing* (1,200-4,000 B.C.), the first written record of Chinese medicine. Therefore, when needles are inserted the auricular points, these will effect the meridians of the body and enhance the therapuetic effect.

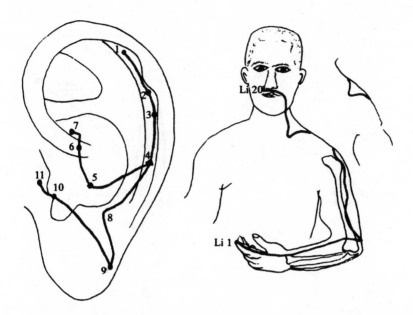

Fig. K-1. The Pathway of the Large Intestine Meridian in the Auricle

1. Starts from fingers
2. wrist
3. elbow
4. shoulder
5. connects to the lung
6. descends to the diaphragm
7. belongs to the large intestine
8. comes from the shoulder and goes up to the neck
9. cheek
10. internal nose
11. external nose

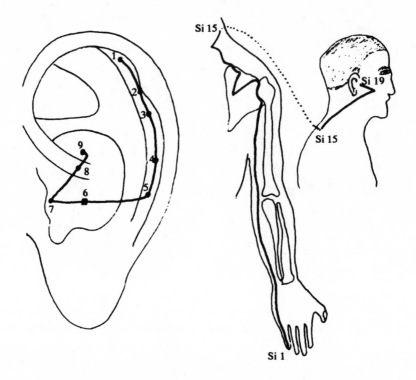

Fig. K–2. Pathway of the Small Intestine Meridian in the Auricle

1. Starts from the fingers
2. wrist
3. elbow
4. shoulder
5. shoulder joint
6. connects to the heart
7. along the pharynx and larynx
8. descends to the diaghragm
9. belongs to the small intestine

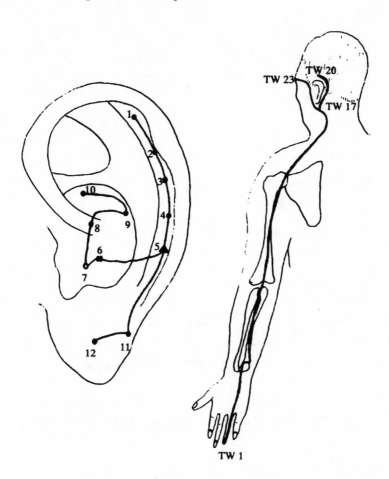

Fig. K–3. The Pathway of the Triple Warmer Meridian in the Auricle

1. Starts from the fingers
2. wrist
3. elbow
4. shoulder
5. shoulder joint
6. connects to the pericardium
7. belongs to the sanjiao
8. go down to the diaphragm
9. pass through to the liver and gall bladder
10. arrive at the urinary bladder
11. comes from the shoulder joint and goes up to internal ear
12. eye

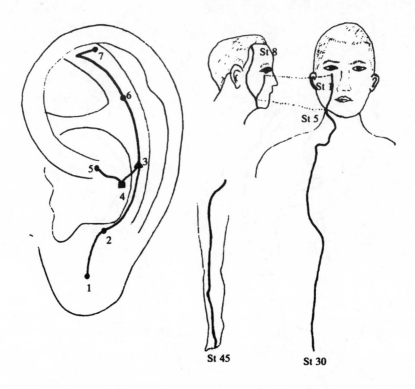

Fig K–4. The Pathway of the Stomach Meridian in the Auricle

1. Starts from the eye
2. head
3. chest
4. connects to the spleen
5. belongs to the stomach
6. knee
7. toes

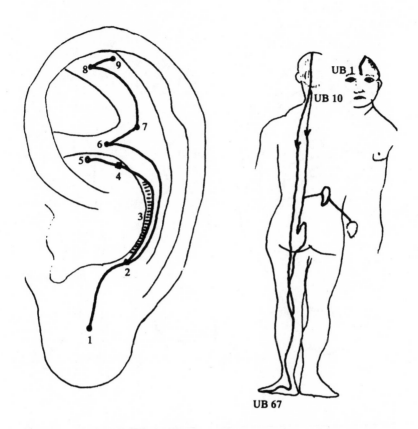

Fig. K–5. The Pathway of the Urinary Bladder Meridian in the Auricle

1. Starts from the eye
2. head
3. along the back
4. connects to the kidney
5. belongs to the urinary bladder
6. comes from head to the buttock
7. knee
8. heel
9. toes

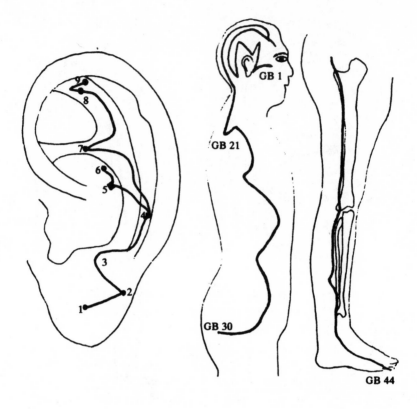

Fig. K–6. The Pathway of the Gall Bladder Meridian in the Auricle

1. Starts from the eye
2. internal ear
3. head
4. along the neck to the shoulder
5. connects to the liver
6. belongs to the gall bladder
7. comes from shoulder to the buttock
8. ankle
9. toes

Chapter XI

Moxibustion

CHAPTER XI. MOXIBUSTION

Moxibustion is a therapeutic technique in which the herb "artemesia vulgaris", or mugwort, is burned on or near the body, usually at acupuncture points. "Moxa", as the herb is known, is a small plant that grows abundantly on mountains and in fields (Fig. 1). The leaves are harvested, dried, pounded and cleaned in a sieve until the rough debris falls away leaving a soft, light colored wool. The more the moxa is cleaned, the purer it becomes and the lighter in color. Good quality moxa will spring back like a sponge when pressed.

"Pure" moxa wool (Fig. 2) of the highest grade is best for use in direct moxa techniques in which the moxa is in contact with the skin. Medium grade moxa is used for warming needle techniques. Coarse moxa is used in moxa poles and for indirect moxa techniques in which there is a medium between the moxa and the skin. Moxa should be stored in a dry container and periodically dried in the sun.

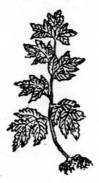

Fig. 1: Moxa plant (Artemesia vulgaris L. var indica Maxim)

Moxibustion produces a penetrating heat and the fire is non-toxic. Moxa has antiseptic properties and was used in ancient times to heal burns. The older the moxa, the stronger are its medicinal properties.

Functions

The technique of moxibustion is commonly used in the treatment of cold patterns of disease which are considered to be a Yin disorder. The nature of moxa is said to be "pure Yang." The heat from moxibustion penetrates deep beneath the skin into the acupuncture point and then into the meridian. Moxibustion has the following functions:

1. Restores weakened Yang and expels Cold and Damp

    a. in chronic weakened conditions where the Yang has
        become exhausted.

    b. cold patterns (Yin disorder).

2. Increases the circulation of qi and bloodletting through the me-
    ridians

    a. "penetrates all the channels"; opens the 12 channels and
        removes obstruction.

    b. promotes the healing of injured muscles.

3. Promotes the normal functioning of the organs

    a. warms the uterus.

    b. "courses through the three yin."

Applications

Moxibustion is indicated in a wide ranges of disorders. The following are examples of the most common clinical applications of moxibustion. This is a brief outline of conditions and is not a full descrip-
tion of the etiology or treatment of these conditions.

Asthma

Etiology: Wind and cold invade the lungs causing obstruction by
phlegm and dampness.

Moxibustion is used between asthma attacks. *Direct moxa* is applied
at GV 14, UB 12, UB 13, CV 17; "grain of wheat" size or small cone,
3-5 times at each point.

Diarrhea

Etiology: Deficient spleen yang or cold or dampness in the spleen.

Direct moxa at St 25, CV 4, CV 8; 5-7 cones at 2 of the 3 points, rotating points used and treating daily or on alternate days.

Arthritis and Rheumatic Pain

Etiology: Circulation of qi and blood through the channels is hindered by wind, cold and/or dampness. Treatment is focused on restoring balance by opening the channels to spread the qi and blood.

For arthritis associated with cold or dampness: a combination of needling and moxibustion is recommended. Select both local and distal points on channels which traverse the area of pain. For chronic cases of cold or damp arthritis: moxibustion should be used daily. Moxibustion is contraindicated for arthritis associated with heat.

Vomiting and Abdominal Pain

Etiology: Obstruction of stomach qi which may arise from cold in the stomach, or phlegm and dampness in the spleen/stomach causes food or liquids to obstruct the stomach.

For deficiency and cold in the spleen/stomach (with symptoms of pain which diminishes with warmth and pressure but increases if cold food or beverages are consumed, vomiting of clear fluids and undigested food, and loose stool): use moxibustion at UB 20 and UB 21 (to warm the middle jiao) and at CV 4 (to warm the Kidney Yang, the basis of the transformative and transportive functions of spleen/stomach). For phlegm and dampness (with symptoms of frothing vomit, dizziness, palpitations, and a lumpy feeling in the chest region): use moxibustion at CV 14 to facilitate movement in the middle jiao and needle St 40 and Sp 9.

Gynecological Disorders

Moxibustion is applicable in a number of gynecological disorders, including irregular menstruation, dysmenorrhea, amenorrhea, leukorrhea and abnormal uterine bleeding. Refer to a text for discussion of specific treatments. For fetus in breach position, warm UB 67 with moxa pole for 30 minutes daily until fetus is correctly positioned. For insufficient lactation due to deficiency of qi and blood or to depressed liver qi causing obstruction, use moxa pole at CV 17 and St 18 for 10-20 minutes; also direct moxa at CV 17 and S.I. 1.

Methods of Application

There are two techniques of moxibustion therapy: direct and indirect moxibustion.

<u>Direct Moxa</u>

Direct moxa involves burning a small piece of moxa wool directly on the skin. There are two methods of direct moxibustion: pustulating (blister-forming) and non-pustulating.

1. Pustulating Method

Small cones of moxa are placed on the skin at the acupuncture point and are burned completely (Fig. 3). This does cause the patient pain. After a few days, a blister forms and must be treated daily with ointment to guard against infection. A small scar will finally replace the blister. Because this method of moxibustion is painful, presents the danger of infection and causes scarring, it is generally not used in clinical practice.

2. Non-Pustulating Method

This method provides strong stimulation without burning the skin, forming a blister or leaving a scar. The burning cone is quickly removed with tweezers when it begins to cause pain but before it burns the skin. Generally, 3-7 cones of moxa wool are applied. This technique is used for mild deficient cold patterns.

A variation of this method is to burn tiny cones, called "grain of wheat" cones, on a thin layer of petroleum jelly. The ointment affixes the moxa at the site and protect the skin from blistering.

Sizes Of Moxa Cones

Sesame Seed
1/2 Rice
Green Beans (Mung)
Red Bean
Yellow Bean (Soy)
1/2 Peanut

To form a moxa cone, place a small amount of moxa wool in your hand and roll it between the first two fingers in one direction. The cone should be round in shape, tight and uniform. When ignited, moxa tends not to crumble but a loosely rolled cone will be less manageable to work with. Rolling the cone in one direction is more effective than rolling it back and forth.

Larger moxa cones may be cone-shaped, or pyramid-shaped. To form them, place the moxa wool into he palm of one hand and pinch it into a cone with the fingers of the other hand so that it is uniform and tight. Smaller cones are used for direct moxa and larger cones are suitable for indirect moxibustion.

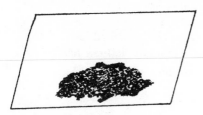

Fig. 2. Moxa wool   .   Fig. 3. Moxa cones

Indirect Moxa

For indirect cauterization, moxa is burned above the skin, on a needle or on a heat-transfer medium.

1. Moxa Sticks

A moxa stick, or moxa pole, is a cigar of the moxa leaves. The moxa pole is lit at one end and is held about 1" above the skin so that the heat warms the area below. The patient is always comfortable and the skin reddens but does not burn or blister. Normally, this requires 5-10 minutes.

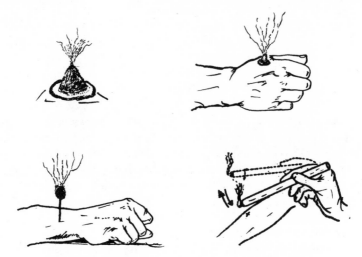

Fig. 4 Methods of moxibustion application

The moxa pole can be moved evenly in a circular pattern to spread the focus of heat over a large area. This is particularly effective where there is pain due to obstruction, soft tissue injuries, and skin disorders. Another method, the "sparrow pecking" method, involves moving the moxa pole up and down at the point to facilitate heat penetration and when strong stimulation is required (see Fig. 4).

2. Warming Needle

There are three warming needle techniques in which the heat from the moxa is transferred to the point through the needle. These are useful when there are many needles to be heated.

a. A 3/4" *slice of the moxa pole* is cut off and is fitted onto the handle of the needle. The slice of moxa is ignited. A small piece of cardboard or tinfoil serving as a skin protector may be placed around the base of the needle to catch any moxa ash that might fall.

   Application: deep pain in the joints; stiff pain in the shoulders and knees; abdominal masses or tumors.

b. A small amount of *moxa wool* is wrapped around the handle and ignited. A skin protector is often used.

Application: cold and dampness in the joints causing pain and stiffness.

c. The moxa stick is held close to the handle of the needle transferring heat to the needle, into the point, and thus into the meridian.

3. Moxa Instrument

A metal container with a screen at the bottom is used to hold loose moxa. The moxa inside is ignited and the instrument held over the pint or moved over a large area until redness appears. A piece of protective gauze may be placed on the skin and the moxa instrument rolled over the CV meridian from CV 3 to CV 8.

4. Heat-Transfer Mediums

With this technique, a medium is placed between the burning moxa and the skin. The medium can be lifted from the skin to control the amount of heat during treatment or to treat two points at the same time. This method is not painful and presents little risk of infection. Several kinds of mediums are used: ginger, garlic, salt, aconite (Fu Zi), pepper and mud plasters.

GINGER: Slice fresh ginger root to a thickness of 0.3 inches (width of two quarters) and perforate it with several holes. Use a large moxa cone. Ginger is a hot herb and the liquid from the root can cause blistering. During treatment, the ginger should be lifted and the skin examined for redness or irritation. A blister can form even though the patient does not feel too much heat at the site (See Fig. 4).

Application: diarrhea due to deficient spleen/stomach; abdominal pain; painful joints; deficient cold conditions in general.

GARLIC: This has the same preparation as for ginger. Garlic has an irritant properly so a blister may form if the moxa is allowed to burn too long. Check for redness and temperature.

Application: scrofula; early stage of skin infections; poisonous insect bites; pulmonary tuberculosis; abdominal masses; non-ulcerated carbuncles.

ACONITE: Aconite is an acrid and hot herb that warms the kidneys and strengthens the Yang. A slice of the aconite root (Aconitum Carmichael) or a paste of ground aconite and yellow wine is placed on the point and moxa is burned on it. *Herb cakes* consisting of aconite and similar hot, aromatic, drying herbs are used as a heat-transfer medium. A thin layer of gauze is sometimes used between the cake and the skin to minimize irritation.

Application: deficient Yang conditions including skin ulcerations that resist healing or Yin abscesses and carbuncles where the pus will not disperse.

PEPPER: A paste is made of white pepper mixed with flour. Powdered herbs such as cinnamon or cloves can be added to the center of the paste.

Application: arthritic pain; local numbness; stiffness.

MUD PLASTERS: Mud is used as a heat-transfer medium for burning moxa.

Application: localized eczema and other skin diseases.

SALT: Salt is used only in the umbilicus. The naval depression is filled with salt and a moxa cone is placed directly on the salt. The salt absorbs the heat from the moxa and warmth spreads slowly outward from CV 8. If the heat becomes too great, the moxa may be removed with forceps and the handle of the forceps may be inserted into the salt. The metal handle will absorb the heat from the salt.

Application: acute abdominal pain accompanied by vomiting and diarrhea, dysentery and collapse with symptoms of cold limbs and no pulse after severe vomiting and diarrhea ("abandoned stroke").

Precautions

1. Avoid inadvertent burns and treat those which do occur.

2. Moxibustion is contraindicated for patients with febrile diseases and must not be used on the lower back or abdomen of pregnant women.

3. Do not use in the areas of the sensory organs or mucous membranes. Direct moxa should not be used on the face, the breast, over large blood vessels, prominent tendons or major creases in the skin.

4. Care must be taken when performing moxibustion over areas of numbness or on patients who are unconscious to avoid too much stimulation.

Chapter XII

Cupping and Gwa Sha Therapies

CHAPTER XII.   CUPPING and GWA SHA THERAPIES

TRADITIONAL CUPPING THERAPY

Cupping is a method of treating disease by causing local congestion. A partial vacuum is created in a jar, or "cup", which s then applied to the skin. The underlying tissue is drawn up into the jar causing blood stasis. Cups are left in place for 5-15 minutes or until there is local congestion. Cupping often leaves a purplish mark that will disappear without special treatment.

Indications

arthritic pain	common cold
indigestion	dysmenorrhea
non-ulcerated furuncle	headache
abdominal pain	eye disorders
cough	stomach-ache
hypertension	low back pain
pertussis in children	poisonous snake bite

Traditional Method

1. Clean the area with alcohol.

2. Hold an alcohol-soaked cotton ball with tweezers and ignite it.

3. With the other hand, hold the cup near the body.

4. Quickly insert the cotton ball into the cup and out again and quickly place the cup onto the body. The flame creates a partial vacuum in the cup which will draw the skin upward into the jar. A good seal is obtained when the cup attaches firmly onto the skin and the suction holds it in place.

5   If applying a second cup, position it at least 5 cm distal to the first.

6. Cups should be left in place until there is local congestion, usually 5-15 minutes.

7. Single cups can be used on smaller areas or at specific points of tenderness; several cups may be used over wider areas such as over a strained muscle.

8. To remove cups, press with a finger on the skin at the base of the cup to break the seal and then lift the cup. Do not try to pull a cup off.

9. Clean the area with alcohol to remove any moisture or blood.

Since some patients are nervous about fire cups, many acupuncturists now use suctions cups instead.

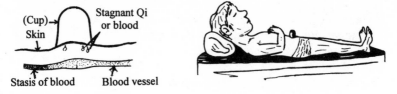

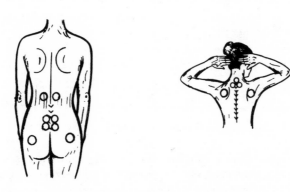

Fig. 1. Methods of cupping application

There are three varieties of cupping:

1. Sliding Cups: This method of cupping is used over large, flat body areas such as the back or thighs. The rim of the cup is lubricated with an oil; the cup is applied; the cup is moved by holding the cup at the base, slightly lifting the front edge in the direction of the movement and pressing the back edge without breaking

the seal. Continue until the skin has reddened. With this technique, avoid bony prominence.

2. Cupping with a Needle: This technique of cupping is often used for treatment of rheumatism and is considered more effective than cupping alone in the treatment of this disease. The point is needled; the qi is obtained; the needle is retained (left in place); the cup is prepared and placed over the needle on the surrounding skin.

3. Cupping with Bloodletting: This method of cupping is used in the treatment of soft tissue injury, neurodermatitis, pruritis, neurasthenia, gastrointestinal nervous dysfunction. First, bleeding is done (or cutaneous acupuncture), then cupping.

Contraindications

Cupping is not indicated in the following situations:

1. In the presence of high fever.

2. If there are convulsions or cramps.

3. For allergic skin conditions or ulcerated sores.

And cupping should not be done in the following areas:

4. Over thin musculature, bony or angular prominence or depressions.

5. On the abdomen or lower back of pregnant women.

TRADITIONAL GWA SHA THERAPY

"Sha" Therapy or "Gwa Sha" is a technique of "scratching" or scraping the skin with a smooth-edged instrument in order to elicit a redness of the skin. "Sha" means "sand" and, in this context, it refers to the sand-like appearance of the skin when scratched. The presence of "sha" indicates stagnation of qi and blood causing local obstruction. A sign of "sha" is that, when the painful muscle is firmly pressed with the thumb, the skin will appear white and will remain this way for a time.

Indications

A sign of "sha" is whiteness of the skin when pressed firmly. The symptoms that indicate "gwa sha" are pain and fatigue in the muscles. "Sha" is often present in people who do a lot of physical labor in their daily life, overworking specific muscle groups and causing muscle contraction and the obstruction of circulation.

Sha Therapy can be used in cases of high fever. Scrape the back downward along both sides of the spine from T 1 to coccyx until skin becomes dark purple. This has a definite effect on lowering fever.

Traditional Methods

1. Clean the area with alcohol.

2. Apply a thin film of oil or ointment (Vaseline) over area to be scraped.

3. Using a smooth-edged instrument (a Chinese porcelain spoon), begin to scrape the skin in a downward movement and in the same direction. Use a firm pressure, increasing slightly as you continue to scrape. Move over different areas of the muscle (angle left, angle right) following the direction of the muscle fibers.

4. Ask the patient how s/he is feeling; the patient should feel comfortable.

5. Look for "sha": "sha" appears as red dots that come up to the surface of the skin as it is scrapped. If there is a lot of "sha", there may appear dark purple or black spots. This will have a beneficial effect on the patient since it will relieve the muscles of the tired, sore feeling that was present.

6. Check that the oil or ointment is still lubricating the skin. Another application of lubricant may be required (but apply thinly). If the oil is scrapped away, the skin will feel pulled and irritated and the patient will feel discomfort.

7. Discontinue treatment when the skin is red or dark.

8. Wipe the area with gauze or cotton and alcohol to both clean the area of oils and disinfect the area.

9. Advise the patient that the redness is normal and should disperse within a day or two. Tell the patient that this is a treatment for tired, sore and painful muscles and that s/he should feel more comfortable. Also advise the patient to avoid starchy, fried (oily) or roasted foods for 24 hours to give the body a chance to heal.

Gwa Sha can be performed in the area of the neck, the back, the arms, the legs, and close to joints which feel tired and painful.

Contraindications

1. Do not scrape directly over joints or bony areas. Scraping is done over muscle fibers. To elicit the "Sha" in the area of a joint, scraping may be done on the tendons surrounding the joint and on their muscles.

2. Do not apply gwa sha over areas of skin that is inflamed (red, hot and swollen), nor over areas of skin that is broken (abrasions, cuts, injuries or sores that are weeping).

APPENDIX

ACUPUNCTURE POINTS

I.   The Lung Meridian of Hand - Taiyin (Lu)

1.	Lu 1	(Zhongfu, Chungfu)
2.	Lu 2	(Yunmen, Yun Men)
3.	Lu 3	(Tianfu, Tien Fu)
4.	Lu 4	(Xiabai, Hsia Pai)
5.	Lu 5	(Chize, Chih Tsen)
6.	Lu 6	(Kongzui, Kon Tsui)
7.	Lu 7	(Lieque, Lieh Chueh)
8.	Lu 8	(Jingqu, Ching Chu)
9.	Lu 9	(Taiyuan, Tai Yuan)
10.	Lu10	(Yuji, Yu Chi)
11.	Lu11	(Shaoshang, Shao Shang)

II. The Large Intestine Meridian of Hand - Yangming (LI)

1.	LI 1	(Shangyang, Shang Yang)
2.	LI 2	(Erjian, Erh Chien)
3.	LI 3	(Sanjian, San Chien)
4.	LI 4	(Hegu, Hoh Ku)
5.	LI 5	(Yangxi, Yang Tsih)
6.	LI 6	(Pianli, Pien Li)
7.	LI 7	(Wenliu, Wen Liu)
8.	LI 8	(Xialian, Hsia Lien)
9.	LI 9	(Shanglian, Shang Lien)
10.	LI10	(Shousanli, Shou San Li)
11.	LI11	(Quchi, Chu Chih)
12.	LI12	(Zhouliao, Chou Liao)
13.	LI13	(Hand - Wuli, Wu Li)
14.	LI14	(Biano, Pi Nao)
15.	LI15	(Jianyu, Chien Yu)
16.	LI16	(Jugu, Chu Ku)
17.	LI17	(Tianding, Tien Ting)
18.	LI18	(Neck - Futu, Fu Tu)
19.	LI19	(Nose - Heliao, Ho Lieo)
20.	LI20	(Yingxiang, Ying Hsiang)

III. The Stomach Meridian of Foot - Yangming (St)

1. St 1 (Chengqi, Cheng Chi)
2. St 2 (Sibai, Ssu Pai)
3. St 3 (Nose - Juliao, Chu Liao)
4. St 4 (Disang, Ti Tsang)
5. St 5 (Daying, Ta Ying)
6. St 6 (Jiache, Chia Tseh)
7. St 7 (Xiaguan, Hsia Kuan)
8. St 8 (Touwei, Tou Wei)
9. St 9 (Renying, Jen Ying)
10. St 10 (Shuitu, Shui Tu)
11. St 11 (Qishe, Chi She)
12. St 12 (Quepen, Chueh Pen)
13. St 13 (Qihu, Chi Hu)
14. St 14 (Kufang, Ku Fang)
15. St 15 (Wuyi, Wu Yi)
16. St 16 (Yingchuang, Ying Chuang)
17. St 17 (Ruzhong, Ju Chung)
18. St 18 (Rugen, Ju Ken)
19. St 19 (Burong, Pu Yung)
20. St 20 (Chengman, Cheng Man)
21. St 21 (Liangmen, Liang Men)
22. St 22 (Guanmen, Kuan Men)
23. St 23 (Taiyi, Tai Yi)
24. St 24 (Huaroumen, Hua Juo Men)
25. St 25 (Tianshu, Tien Shu)
26. St 26 (Wailing Wei Ling)
27. St 27 (Daju, Ta Chu)
28. St 28 (Shuidao, Shui Tao)
29. St 29 (Guilai, Kuei Lai)
30. St 30 (Qichong, Chi Chung)
31. St 31 (Biguan, Pi Kuan)
32. St 32 (Futu, Fu Tu)
33. St 33 (Yinshi, Yin Shih)
34. St 34 (Liangqui, Liang Chiu)
35. St 35 (Dubi, Tu Pi)
36. St 36 (Zusanli, Tsu San Li)
37. St 37 (Shangjuxu, Shang Chu Hsu)
38. St 38 (Tiaokou, Tiao Kou)
39. St 39 (Xiajuxu, Hsia Chu Hsu)

40.	St 40	(Fenglong, Feng Lung)
41.	St 41	(Jiexi, Chieh Tsi)
42.	St 42	(Chungyang, Chung Yang)
43.	St 43	(Xiangu, Hsien Ku)
44.	St 44	(Neiting, Nei Ting)
45.	St 45	(Lidui, Li Tui)

IV. The Spleen Meridian of Foot - Taiyin (Sp)

1.	Sp 1	(Yinbai, Yin Pai)
2.	Sp 2	(Dadu, Ta Tu)
3.	Sp 3	(Taibai, Tai Pai)
4.	Sp 4	(Gongsun, Kung Sun)
5.	Sp 5	(Shangqiu, Shang Chiu)
6.	Sp 6	(Sanyinjiao, San Yin Chiao)
7.	Sp 7	(Lougu, Lou Ku)
8.	Sp 8	(Diji, Ti Chi)
9.	Sp 9	(Yinlingquan, Yin Ling Chuan)
10.	Sp 10	(Xuehai, Hsuen Hai)
11.	Sp 11	(Jimen, Chi Men)
12.	Sp 12	(Chongmen, Chung Men)
13.	Sp 13	(Fushe, Fu She)
14.	Sp 14	(Fujie, Fu Chieh)
15.	Sp 15	(Daheng, Ta Heng)
16.	Sp 16	(Fuai, Fu Ai)
17.	Sp 17	(Shidou, Shih Tou)
18.	Sp 18	(Tianxi, Tien Tsih)
19.	Sp 19	(Xiongxiang, Hsiung Hsia)
20.	Sp 20	(Zhourong, Chou Yung)
21.	Sp 21	(Dabao, Ta Pao)

V. The Heart Meridian of Hand - Shaoyin (Ht)

1.	Ht 1	(Jiquan, Chi Chuan)
2.	Ht 2	(Qingling, Ching Ling)
3.	Ht 3	(Shaohai, Shao Hai)
4.	Ht 4	(Lingdao, Ling Tao)
5.	Ht 5	(Tongli, Tung Li)
6.	Ht 6	(Yinxi, Yin Hsi)
7.	Ht 7	(Shenmen, Shen Men)
8.	Ht 8	(Shaofu, Shao Fu)
9.	Ht 9	(Shaochong, Shao Chung)

VI. The Small Intestine Meridian of Hand - Taiyang (SI)

1. SI 1   (Shaoze, Shao Tse)
2. SI 2   (Qiangu, Chien Ku)
3. SI 3   (Houxi, Hou Hsi)
4. SI 4   (Wangu, Wan Ku)
5. SI 5   (Yanggu, Yang Ku)
6. SI 6   (Yanglao, Yang Lao)
7. SI 7   (Zhizheng, Chi Cheng)
8. SI 8   (Xiaohai, Hsiao Hai)
9. SI 9   (Jianzhen, Chien Chin)
10. SI 10   (Naoshu, Nao Yu)
11. SI 11   (Tianzong, Tien Tsung)
12. SI 12   (Bingfeng, Ping Feng)
13. SI 13   (Quyuan, Chu Huan)
14. SI 14   (Jianwaishu, Chien Wai Yu)
15. SI 15   (Jianzhongshu, Chien Chung Yu)
16. SI 16   (Tianchuang, Tien Chuan)
17. SI 17   (Tianrong, Tien Yung)
18. SI 18   (Quanliao, Chuan Liao)
19. SI 19   (Tinggong , Ting Kung)

VII. The Urinary Bladder Meridian of Foot - Taiyang (UB)

1. UB 1   (Jingming, Ching Ming)
2. UB 2   (Zanzhu, Tsuan Chu)
3. UB 3   (Miechong, Mei Chung)
4. UB 4   (Quchai, Chu Cha)
5. UB 5   (Wuchu, Wu Chu)
6. UB 6   (Chengquang, Cheng Kuang)
7. UB 7   (Tontiang Tung Tien)
8. UB 8   (Luoque, Lo Chueh)
9. UB 9   (Yuzhen, Yu Chin)
10. UB 10   (Tianzhu, Tien Chu)
11. UB 11   (Dashu, Ta Chu)
12. UB 12   (Fengmen, Feng Men)
13. UB 13   (Feishu, Fei Yu)
14. UB 14   (Jueyinshu, Chuen Yin Yu)
15. UB 15   (Xinshu, Hsin Yu)
16. UB 16   (Dushu, Tu Yu)
17. UB 17   (Geshu, Keh Yu)

18.	UB 18	(Ganshu, Kan Yu)
19.	UB 19	(Danshu, Tan Yu)
20.	UB 20	(Pishu Pi Yu)
21.	UB 21	(Weishu, Wei Yu)
22.	UB 22	(Sanjiaoshu, San Chiao Yu)
23.	UB 23	(Shenshu, Shen Yu)
24.	UB 24	(Qihaishu, Chi Hai Yu)
25.	UB 25	(Dachangshu, Ta Chang Yu)
26.	UB 26	(Guanyuanshu, Kuan Chang Yu)
27.	UB 27	(Xiaochangshu, Hsiao Chang Yu)
28.	UB 28	(Pangguangshu, Pang Kuang Yu)
29.	UB 29	(Zhonglushu, Chung Lu Yu)
30.	UB 30	(Baihuanshu, Pai Huan Yu)
31.	UB 31	(Shangliao, Shang Liao)
32.	UB 32	(Ciliao, Tzu Liao)
33.	UB 33	(Zhongliao, Chung Liao)
34.	UB 34	(Xialiao, Hsio Liao)
35.	UB 35	(Huiyang, Hui Yang)
36.	UB 36	(Fufen, Fu Fen)
37.	UB 37	(Pohu, Pai Hu)
38.	UB 38	(Gaohuangshu, Kao Huang)
39.	UB 39	(Shentang, Shen Tang)
40.	UB 40	(Yixi, Yi Hsi)
41.	UB 41	(Geguan, Keh Kuan)
42.	UB 42	(Hunmen, Huen Men)
43.	UB 43	(Yanggang, Yang Kang)
44.	UB 44	(Yishe, Yi She)
45.	UB 45	(Weicang, Wei Tsang)
46.	UB 46	(Huangmen, Huang Men)
47.	UB 47	(Zhishi, Chi Shih)
48.	UB 48	(Baohuang, Po Huang)
49.	UB 49	(Zhibian, Chi Pien)
50.	UB 50	(Chengfu, Cheng Fu)
51.	UB 51	(Yinmen, Yin Men)
52.	UB 52	(Fuxi, Fu Hsi)
53.	UB 53	(Weiyang, Wei Yang)
54.	UB 54	(Weizhong, Wei Chung)
55.	UB 55	(Heyang, Ho Yang)
56.	UB 56	(Chengjin, Cheng Chin)
57.	UB 57	(Chengshan, Cheng Shan)
58.	UB 58	(Feiyang, Fei Yang)

59. UB 59 (Fuyang, Fu Yang)
60. UB 60 (Kunlun, Kun Lun)
61. UB 61 (Pushen, Pu Shen)
62. UB 62 (Shenmai, Shen Mai)
63. UB 63 (Jinmen, Chin Men)
64. UB 64 (Jinggu, Ching Ku)
65. UB 65 (Shugu, Shu Ku)
66. UB 66 (Tonggu, Tung Ku)
67. UB 67 (Zhiyin, Chi Yin)

VIII. The Kidney Meridian of Foot - Shaoyin (Ki)

1.   Ki 1   (Yongquan, Yung Chuan)
2.   Ki 2   (Rangu, Jan Ku)
3.   Ki 3   (Taixi, Tai Hsi)
4.   Ki 4   (Dazhong, Ta Chung)
5.   Ki 5   (Shuiquan, Shui Chuan)
6.   Ki 6   (Zhaohai, Chao Hai)
7.   Ki 7   (Fuliu, Fu Liu)
8.   Ki 8   (Jiaoxin, Chiao Hsin)
9.   Ki 9   (Zhubin, Chu Pin)
10. Ki 10 (Yingu, Yin Ku)
11. Ki 11 (Henggu, Heng Ku)
12. Ki 12 (Dahe, Ta Hoh)
13. Ki 13 (Quixue, Chi Hsueh)
14. Ki 14 (Siman, Ssu Man)
15. Ki 15 (Zhongzhu, Chung Chu)
16. Ki 16 (Huangshu, Huang Yu)
17. Ki 17 (Shangqu, Shang Chu)
18. Ki 18 (Shiguan Shih Kuan)
19. Ki 19 (Yindu, Yin Tu)
20. Ki 20 (Tonggu, Tung Ku)
21. Ki 21 (Youmen, Yiu Men)
22. Ki 22 (Bulang, Pu Lang)
23. Ki 23 (Shenfen, Shen Feng)
24. Ki 24 (Lingxu, Ling Hsu)
25. Ki 25 (Shencang, Shen Tsang)
26. Ki 26 (Yuzhong, Yu Chung)
27. Ki 27 (Shufu, Yu Fu)

IX. The Pericardium Meridian of Hand - Jueyin (Pc)

1. Pc 1 (Tianchi, Tien Chih)
2. Pc 2 (Tianquan, Tien Chuan)
3. Pc 3 (Quze, Chu Tseh)
4. Pc 4 (Ximen, Hsi Men)
5. Pc 5 (Jianshi, Chien Shi)
6. Pc 6 (Neiguan, Nei Kuan)
7. Pc 7 (Daling, Ta Ling)
8. Pc 8 (Laogong, Lao Kung)
9. Pc 9 (Zhongchong, Chung Chung)

X. The Triple Warmer Meridian of Hand - Shaoyang (TW)

1. TW 1 (Guanchong, Kuan Chung)
2. TW 2 (Yemen, Yeh Men)
3. TW 3 (Zhongzhu, Chung Tu)
4. TW 4 (Yangchi, Yang Chih)
5. TW 5 (Waiguan, Wai Kuan)
6. TW 6 (Zhigou, Chih Kou)
7. TW 7 (Huizong, Hui Tsung)
8. TW 8 (Sanyangluo, San Yang Lo)
9. TW 9 (Sidu, Ssu Tu)
10. TW 10 (Tianjing, Tien Ching)
11. TW 11 (Qinglengyuan, Ching Leng Yuan)
12. TW 12 (Xiaoluo, Siao Lo)
13. TW 13 (Naohui, Nao Hui)
14. TW 14 (Jianliao, Chieh Liao)
15. TW 15 (Tranliao, Tien Liao)
16. TW 16 (Tranyou,Tien Hu)
17. TW 17 (Yifeng Yi Feng)
18. TW 18 (Qimai, Chi Mo)
19. TW 19 (Luxi, Lu Hsi)
20. TW 20 (Jiaosun, Chiao, Sun)
21. TW 21 (Ermen, Erh Men)
22. TW 22 (Heliao, Ho Liao)
23. TW 23 (Sizhukong, Ssu Chu Kung)

XI. The Gallbladder Meridian of Foot - Shaoyang (GB)

1. GB 1 (Tongziliao, Tung Tsu Liao)

2.   GB 2   (Tinghui, Ting Hui)
3.   GB 3   (Shangguan, Shang Kuan)
4.   GB 4   (Hanyan, Han Yen)
5.   GB 5   (Xuanlu Hsuan Lu)
6.   GB 6   (Xuanli, Hsuan Li)
7.   GB 7   (Qubin, Chuh Pin)
8.   GB 8   (Shuaigu, Shuai Ku)
9.   GB 9   (Tianchong, Tien Chung)
10. GB 10   (Fubai, Fu Pai)
11. GB 11   (Qiaogin, Chiao Yin)
12. GB 12   (Wangu, Wan Ku)
13. GB 13   (Benshen, Pen Shen)
14. GB 14   (Yangbai, Yang Pai)
15. GB 15   (Linqi, Lin Chi)
16. GB 16   (Muchuang, Mu Chuang)
17. GB 17   (Zhengying, Cheng Ying)
18. GB 18   (Chengling, Cheng Ling)
19. GB 19   (Naong, Nao Kung)
20. GB 20   (Fengchi, Feng Chih)
21. GB 21   (Jianjing, Chien Ching)
22. GB 22   (Yuanye, Yuan Yeh)
23. GB 23   (Zhejin, Tsueh Chin)
24. GB 24   (Riyue, Jeh Yueh)
25. GB 25   (Jingmen, Ching Men)
26. GB 26   (Dai mai, Tai Mo)
27. GB 27   (Wushu, Wu Shu)
28. GB 28   (Weidao, Wei Tao)
29. GB 29   (Juliao, Chu Liao)
30. GB 30   (Huantiao, Huan Tiao)
31. GB 31   (Fengshi, Feng Shih)
32. GB 32   (Zhongdu, Chung Tu)
33. GB 33   (Xiyangguan, Yang Kuan)
34. GB 34   (Yanglingquan, Yang Ling Chuan)
35. GB 35   (Yangjiao,Yang Chiao)
36. GB 36   (Waiqiu, Wai Chiu)
37. GB 37   (Guangming, Kuang Ming)
38. GB 38   (Yangfu, Yang Pu)
39. GB 39   (Xuanzhong, Hsuan Chung)
40. GB 40   (Qiuxu, Chiu Hsu)
41. GB 41   (Linqi, Lin Chih)
42. GB 42   (Diwuhui, Ti Wu Hui)

43.   GB 43   (Xiaxi, Hsia Hsi)
44.   GB 44   (Qiaoyin, Chi Yin)

XII. The Liver Meridian of Foot - Jueyin (Liv)

1.   Liv 1   (Dadun, Ta Tun)
2.   Liv 2   (Xingjian, Hsing Chien)
3.   Liv 3   (Taichong, Tai Chung)
4.   Liv 4   (Zhongfeng, Chung Feng)
5.   Liv 5   (Ligou, Li Kou)
6.   Liv 6   (Zhongdu, Chung Tu)
7.   Liv 7   (Xiguan, Hsi Kuan)
8.   Liv 8   (Ququan, Chu Chuan)
9.   Liv 9   (Yinbao, Yin Pao)
10.   Liv 10 (Wuli, Wu Li)
11.   Liv 11 (Yinlian, Yin Lien)
12.   Liv 12 (Jimai, Chi Mo)
13.   Liv 13 (Zhangmen, Chang Men)
14.   Liv 14 (Qimen, Chi Men)

XIII. The Conception Vessel Meridian (CV)

1.   CV 1   (Huiyin, Hui Yin)
2.   CV 2   (Qugu, Chu Ku)
3.   CV 3   (Zhongji, Chung Chi)
4.   CV 4   (Guanyuan, Kuan Yuan)
5.   CV 5   (Shimen, Shih Men)
6.   CV 6   (Qihai, Chi Hai)
7.   CV 7   (Yinjiao, Yin Chiao)
8.   CV 8   (Shenque, Shen Chueh)
9.   CV 9   (Shuifen, Shui Feng)
10.   CV 10 (Xiawan, Hsia Wan)
11.   CV 11 (Jianli, Chien Li)
12.   CV 12 (Zhongwan, Chung Wan)
13.   CV 13 (Shangwan, Shang Wan)
14.   CV 14 (Juque, Chu Chueh)
15.   CV 15 (Jiuwi, Chiu, Wei)
16.   CV 16 (Zhongting, Chung Ting)
17.   CV 17 (Shanzhong, Tan Chung)
18.   CV 18 (Yutang, Yu Tang)
19.   CV 19 (Zigong, Tsu Kung)

20. CV 20   (Huagai, Hua Kai)
21. CV 21   (Xuanji, Hsuan Chi)
22. CV 22   (Tiantu, Tien Tu)
23. CV 23   (Lianquan, Lieh Chuan)
24. CV 24   (Chengjiang, Cheng Chiang)

XIV.   The Governor Vessel Meridian (GV)

1. GV 1   (Changqiang, Chang Chiang)
2. GV 2   (Yaoshu, Yao Yu)
3. GV 3   (Yaoyangguan, Yang Kuan)
4. GV 4   (Mingmen, Ming Men)
5. GV 5   (Xuanshu, Hsuan Shu)
6. GV 6   (Jizhong, Chichung)
7. GV 7   (Zhongshu, Chung Shu)
8. GV 8   (Jinsuo, Chin So)
9. GV 9   (Zhiyang, Chi Yang)
10. GV 10   (Lingtai, Ling Tai)
11. GV 11   (Shendao, Shen Tao)
12. GV 12   (Shenzhu, Shen Chu)
13. GV 13   (Taodao, Tao Tao)
14. GV 14   (Dazhui, Ta Chui)
15. GV 15   (Yamen, Ya Men)
16. GV 16   (Fengfu, Feng Fu)
17. GV 17   (Naohu, Nao Hu)
18. GV 18   (Qiangjian, Chiang Chien)
19. GV 19   (Houding, Huo Ting)
20. GV 20   (Baihui, Pai Hui)
21. GV 21   (Qianding, Chien Ting)
22. GV 22   (Xinhui, Tsung Hui)
23. GV 23   (Shangxing, Shang Hsing)
24. GV 24   (Shenting, Shen Ting)
25. GV 25   (Suliao, Su Liao)
26. GV 26   (Renzhong, Shui Kou)
27. GV 27   (Duiduan, Tui Tung)
28. GV 28   (Yinjiao, Ying Chiao)

ROUTES OF THE TWELVE MERIDIANS
AND EXTRA MERIDIANS
&
POINTS ON THE FOURTEEN MERIDIANS

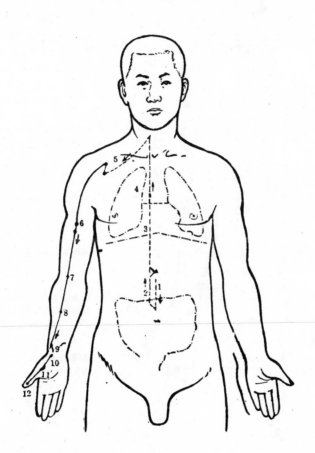

1. Route of the Lung Meridian

442

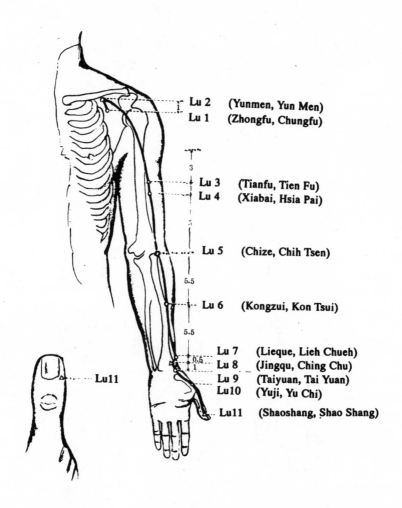

Lu 2 (Yunmen, Yun Men)
Lu 1 (Zhongfu, Chungfu)

3

Lu 3 (Tianfu, Tien Fu)
Lu 4 (Xiabai, Hsia Pai)

Lu 5 (Chize, Chih Tsen)

5.5

Lu 6 (Kongzui, Kon Tsui)

5.5

Lu 7 (Lieque, Lieh Chueh)
Lu 8 (Jingqu, Ching Chu)
Lu 9 (Taiyuan, Tai Yuan)
Lu10 (Yuji, Yu Chi)

Lu11

Lu11 (Shaoshang, Shao Shang)

Points on the Lung Meridian (Lu) - Taiyin

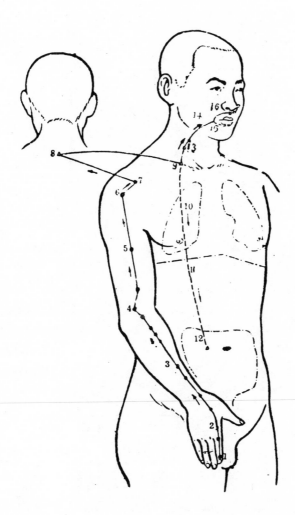

2. Route of the Large Intestine Meridian

444

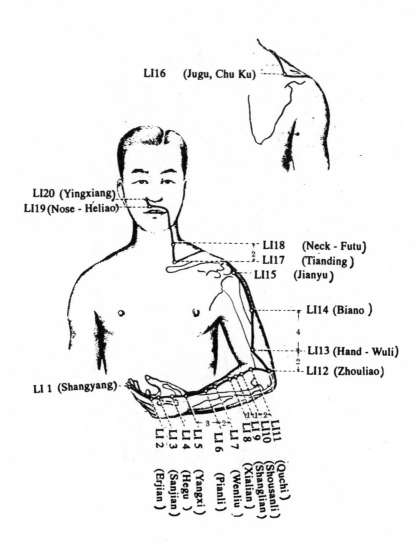

Points on the Large Intestine Meridian (L.I.) - Yangming

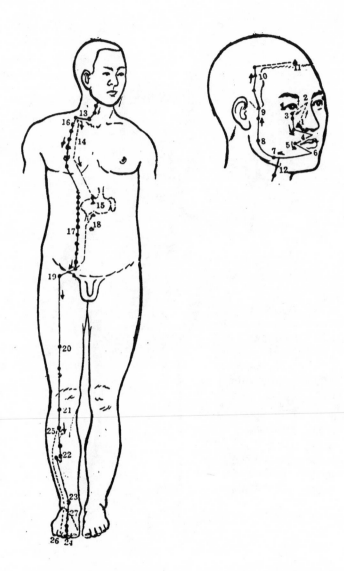

3. Route of the Stomach Meridian

446

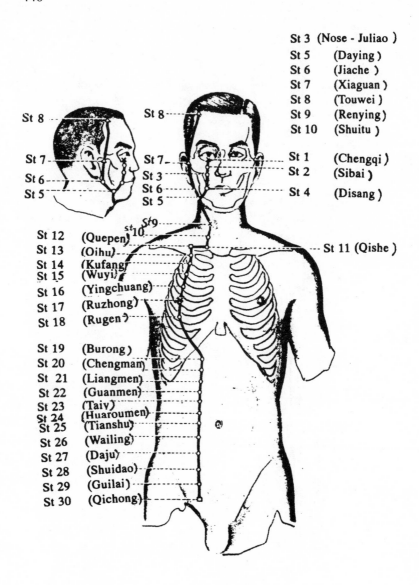

St 3	(Nose - Juliao)
St 5	(Daying)
St 6	(Jiache)
St 7	(Xiaguan)
St 8	(Touwei)
St 9	(Renying)
St 10	(Shuitu)

St 1	(Chengqi)
St 2	(Sibai)
St 4	(Disang)

St 8

St 7
St 6
St 5

St 8
St 7
St 3
St 6
St 5

St 9
St 10

St 11 (Qishe)

St 12	(Quepen)
St 13	(Oihu)
St 14	(Kufang)
St 15	(Wuyi)
St 16	(Yingchuang)
St 17	(Ruzhong)
St 18	(Rugen)
St 19	(Burong)
St 20	(Chengman)
St 21	(Liangmen)
St 22	(Guanmen)
St 23	(Taiv)
St 24	(Huaroumen)
St 25	(Tianshu)
St 26	(Wailing)
St 27	(Daju)
St 28	(Shuidao)
St 29	(Guilai)
St 30	(Qichong)

Points on the Stomach Meridian (St) – Yangming … (1)

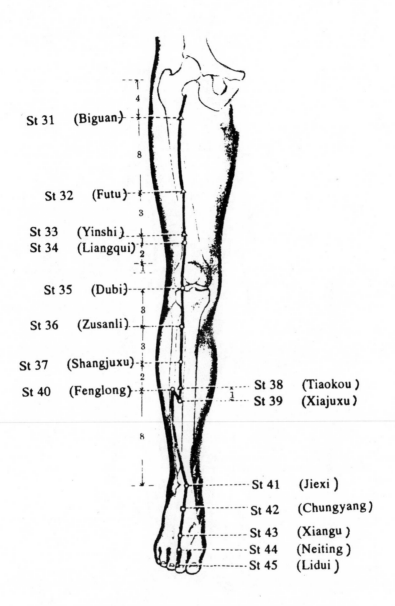

St 31 (Biguan)

St 32 (Futu)

St 33 (Yinshi)
St 34 (Liangqui)

St 35 (Dubi)

St 36 (Zusanli)

St 37 (Shangjuxu)

St 40 (Fenglong)

St 38 (Tiaokou)
St 39 (Xiajuxu)

St 41 (Jiexi)

St 42 (Chungyang)

St 43 (Xiangu)
St 44 (Neiting)
St 45 (Lidui)

Points on the Stomach Meridian (St) – Yangming ... (2)

448

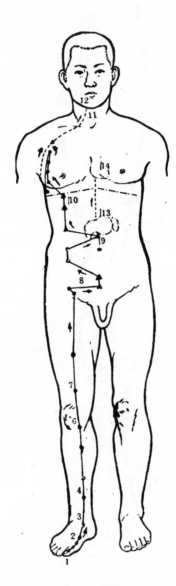

4. Route of the Spleen Meridian

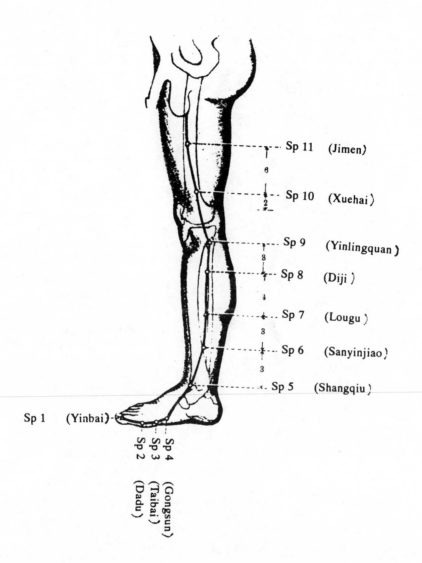

Sp 11   (Jimen)

Sp 10   (Xuehai)

Sp 9   (Yinlingquan)

Sp 8   (Diji)

Sp 7   (Lougu)

Sp 6   (Sanyinjiao)

Sp 5   (Shangqiu)

Sp 1   (Yinbai)

Sp 2   (Dadu)
Sp 3   (Taibai)
Sp 4   (Gongsun)

Points on the Spleen Meridian (Sp) – Taiyin ... (1)

450

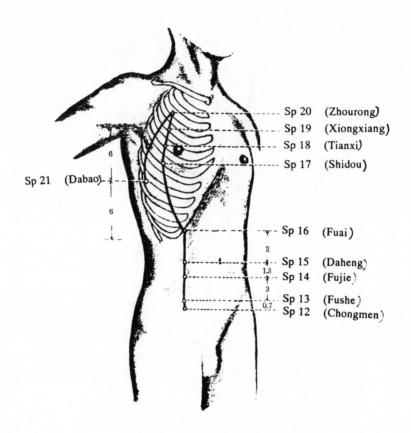

Points on the Spleen Meridian (Sp) – Taiyin ... (2)

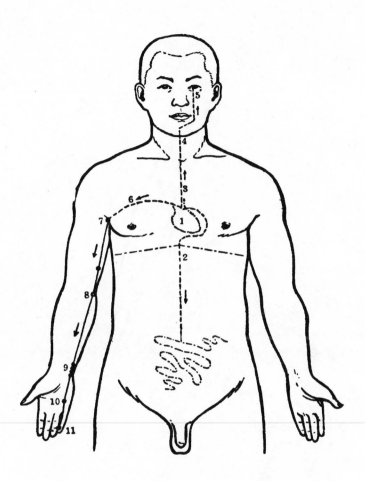

5. Route of the Heart Meridian

452

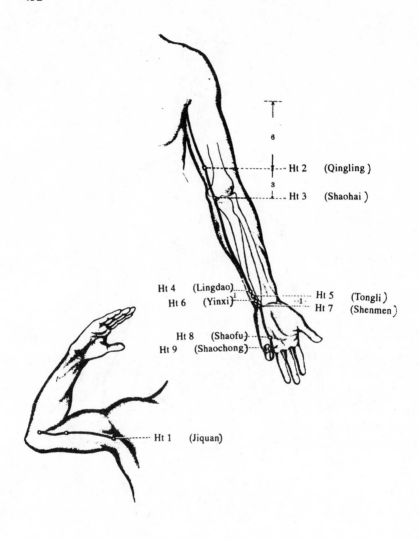

Ht 2   (Qingling)

Ht 3   (Shaohai)

Ht 4   (Lingdao)

Ht 6   (Yinxi)

Ht 5   (Tongli)

Ht 7   (Shenmen)

Ht 8   (Shaofu)

Ht 9   (Shaochong)

Ht 1   (Jiquan)

Points on the Heart Meridian (Ht) – Shaoyin

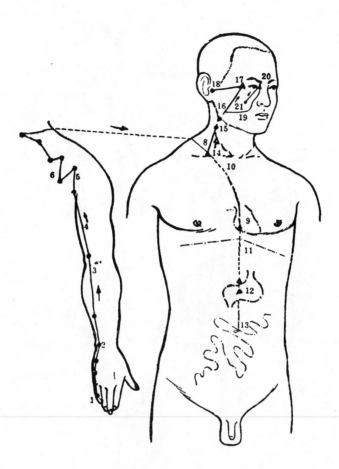

6. Route of the Small Intestines Meridian

454

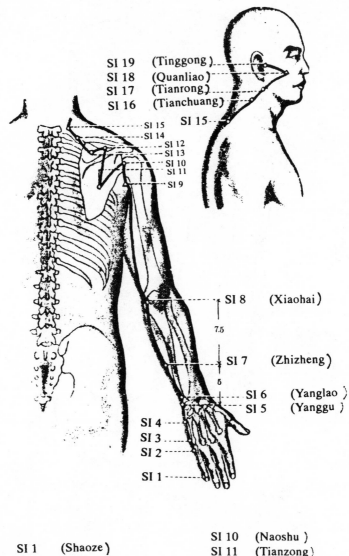

SI 19   (Tinggong)
SI 18   (Quanliao)
SI 17   (Tianrong)
SI 16   (Tianchuang)

SI 15

SI 15
SI 14
SI 12
SI 13
SI 10
SI 11
SI 9

SI 8   (Xiaohai)

7.5

SI 7   (Zhizheng)

5

SI 6   (Yanglao)
SI 5   (Yanggu)

SI 4
SI 3
SI 2

SI 1

SI 1	(Shaoze)	SI 10	(Naoshu)
SI 2	(Qiangu)	SI 11	(Tianzong)
SI 3	(Houx)	SI 12	(Bingfeng)
SI 4	(Wangu)	SI 13	(Quyuan)
SI 9	(Jianzhen)	SI 14	(Jianwaishu)
		SI 15	(Jianzhongshu)

Points on the Small Intestines (S.I.) – Taiying

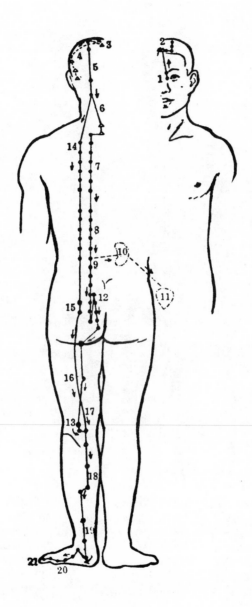

7. Route of the Urinary Bladder Meridian

456

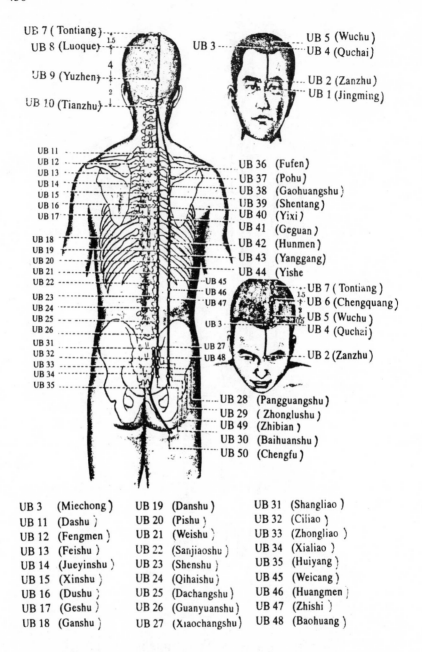

UB 7 (Tontiang)
UB 8 (Luoque)
UB 9 (Yuzhen)
UB 10 (Tianzhu)

UB 3
UB 5 (Wuchu)
UB 4 (Quchai)
UB 2 (Zanzhu)
UB 1 (Jingming)

UB 11
UB 12
UB 13
UB 14
UB 15
UB 16
UB 17
UB 18
UB 19
UB 20
UB 21
UB 22
UB 23
UB 24
UB 25
UB 26
UB 31
UB 32
UB 33
UB 34
UB 35

UB 36 (Fufen)
UB 37 (Pohu)
UB 38 (Gaohuangshu)
UB 39 (Shentang)
UB 40 (Yixi)
UB 41 (Geguan)
UB 42 (Hunmen)
UB 43 (Yanggang)
UB 44 (Yishe
UB 45
UB 46
UB 47

UB 7 (Tontiang)
UB 6 (Chengquang)
UB 5 (Wuchu)
UB 4 (Quchai)
UB 2 (Zanzhu)

UB 3
UB 27
UB 48

UB 28 (Pangguangshu)
UB 29 (Zhonglushu)
UB 49 (Zhibian)
UB 30 (Baihuanshu)
UB 50 (Chengfu)

UB 3	(Miechong)	UB 19	(Danshu)	UB 31	(Shangliao)
UB 11	(Dashu)	UB 20	(Pishu)	UB 32	(Ciliao)
UB 12	(Fengmen)	UB 21	(Weishu)	UB 33	(Zhongliao)
UB 13	(Feishu)	UB 22	(Sanjiaoshu)	UB 34	(Xialiao)
UB 14	(Jueyinshu)	UB 23	(Shenshu)	UB 35	(Huiyang)
UB 15	(Xinshu)	UB 24	(Qihaishu)	UB 45	(Weicang)
UB 16	(Dushu)	UB 25	(Dachangshu)	UB 46	(Huangmen)
UB 17	(Geshu)	UB 26	(Guanyuanshu)	UB 47	(Zhishi)
UB 18	(Ganshu)	UB 27	(Xiaochangshu)	UB 48	(Baohuang)

Points on the Urinary Bladder Meridian (UB) – Taiying ... (1)

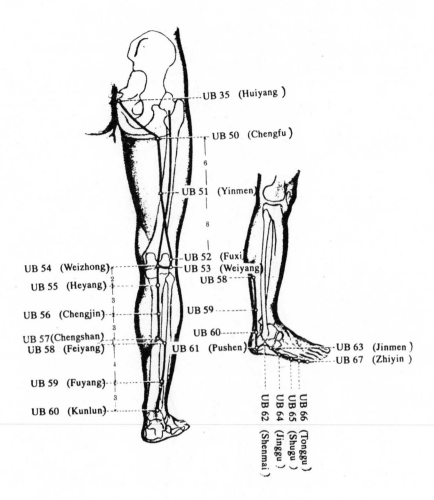

UB 35 (Huiyang)

UB 50 (Chengfu)

6

UB 51 (Yinmen)

8

UB 52 (Fuxi)

UB 54 (Weizhong) ---- UB 53 (Weiyang)

UB 55 (Heyang) ---- UB 58

UB 56 (Chengjin) --- UB 59

UB 57 (Chengshan) --- UB 60

UB 58 (Feiyang) --- UB 61 (Pushen)

UB 59 (Fuyang) ---

UB 60 (Kunlun) ---

UB 63 (Jinmen)

UB 67 (Zhiyin)

UB 62 (Shenmai)
UB 64 (Jinggu)
UB 65 (Shugu)
UB 66 (Tonggu)

Points on the Urinary Bladder Meridian (UB) – Taiying ... (2)

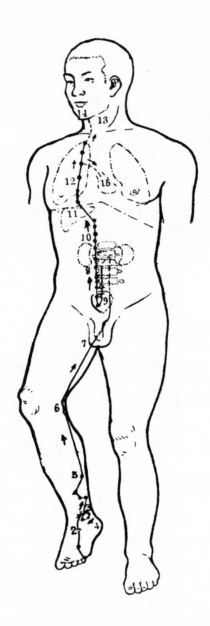

8. Route of the Kidney Meridian

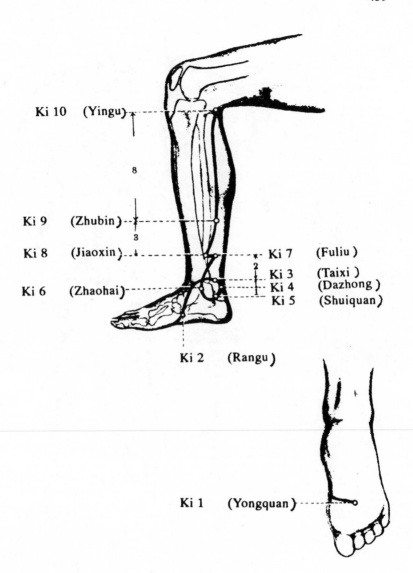

Ki 10 (Yingu)

8

Ki 9 (Zhubin)

3

Ki 8 (Jiaoxin) — Ki 7 (Fuliu)

2
Ki 3 (Taixi)
Ki 4 (Dazhong)
Ki 6 (Zhaohai) — Ki 5 (Shuiquan)

Ki 2 (Rangu)

Ki 1 (Yongquan)

Points on the Kidney Meridian (Ki) – Shayoin ... (1)

460

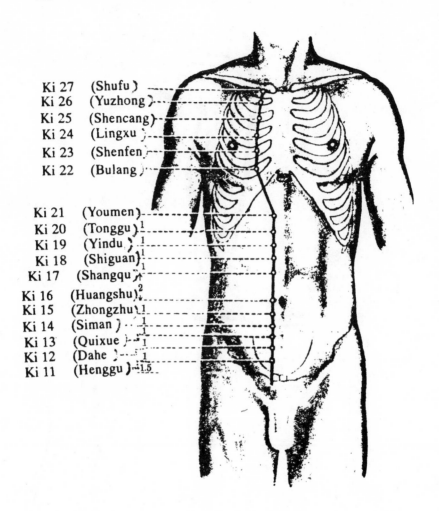

Ki 27   (Shufu)
Ki 26   (Yuzhong)
Ki 25   (Shencang)
Ki 24   (Lingxu)
Ki 23   (Shenfen)
Ki 22   (Bulang)

Ki 21   (Youmen)
Ki 20   (Tonggu)^1
Ki 19   (Yindu)^1
Ki 18   (Shiguan)^1
Ki 17   (Shangqu)^1
Ki 16   (Huangshu)^2
Ki 15   (Zhongzhu)^1
Ki 14   (Siman)^1
Ki 13   (Quixue)^1
Ki 12   (Dahe)^1
Ki 11   (Henggu)$^{1.5}$

Points on the Kidney Meridian (Ki) – Shaoyin … (2)

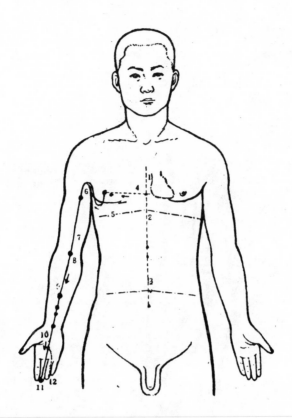

9. Route of the Pericardium Meridian

462

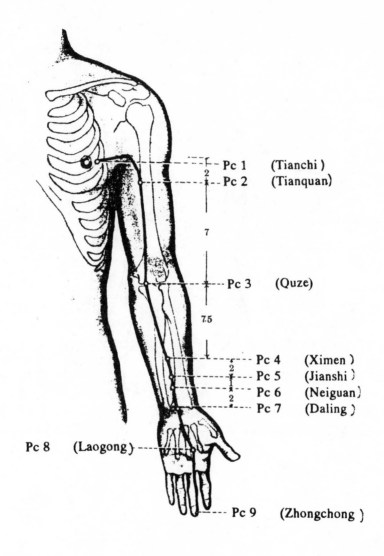

Pc 1 (Tianchi)
Pc 2 (Tianquan)
2
7
Pc 3 (Quze)
7.5
Pc 4 (Ximen)
2
Pc 5 (Jianshi)
Pc 6 (Neiguan)
2
Pc 7 (Daling)
Pc 8 (Laogong)
Pc 9 (Zhongchong)

Points on the Pericardium Meridian (Pc) – Jueyin

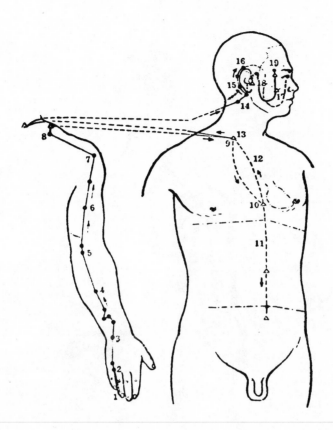

10. Route of the Triple Warmer Meridian

464

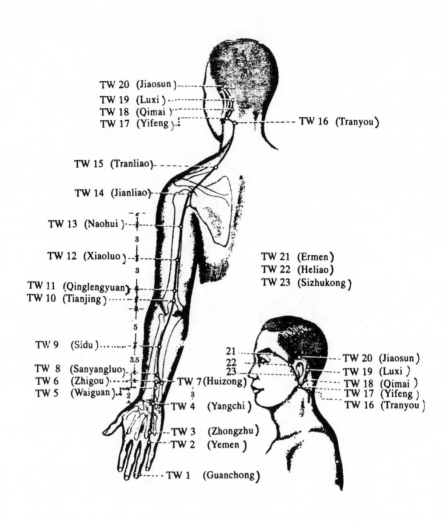

TW 20 (Jiaosun)

TW 19 (Luxi)

TW 18 (Qimai)

TW 17 (Yifeng)

TW 16 (Tranyou)

TW 15 (Tranliao)

TW 14 (Jianliao)

TW 13 (Naohui)

3

TW 12 (Xiaoluo)

3

TW 11 (Qinglengyuan)

TW 10 (Tianjing)

5

TW 9 (Sidu)

3.5

TW 8 (Sanyangluo)

TW 6 (Zhigou)

TW 5 (Waiguan)

2

TW 7 (Huizong)

3

TW 4 (Yangchi)

TW 3 (Zhongzhu)

TW 2 (Yemen)

TW 1 (Guanchong)

TW 21 (Ermen)

TW 22 (Heliao)

TW 23 (Sizhukong)

21

22

23

TW 20 (Jiaosun)

TW 19 (Luxi)

TW 18 (Qimai)

TW 17 (Yifeng)

TW 16 (Tranyou)

Points on the Triple Warmer Meridian (TW) – Shaoyang

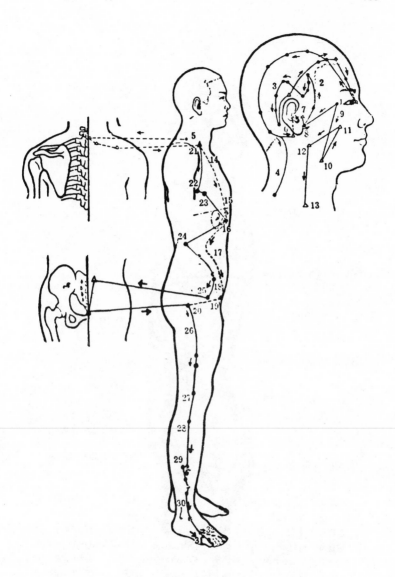

11. Route of the Gall Bladder Meridian

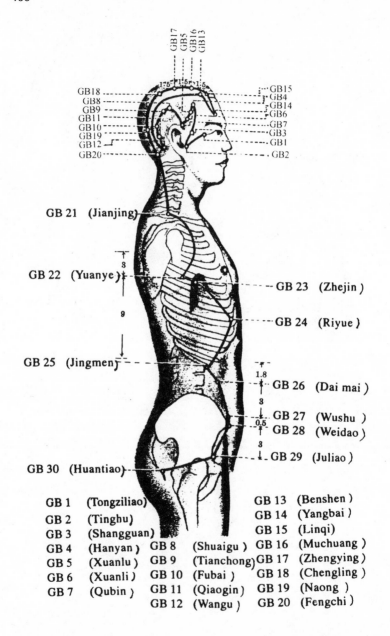

GB17 GB5 GB16 GB13

GB18
GB8
GB9
GB11
GB10
GB19
GB12
GB20

GB15
GB4
GB14
GB6
GB7
GB3
GB1
GB2

GB 21 (Jianjing)

GB 22 (Yuanye)

GB 23 (Zhejin)

GB 24 (Riyue)

GB 25 (Jingmen)

GB 26 (Dai mai)

GB 27 (Wushu)

GB 28 (Weidao)

GB 29 (Juliao)

GB 30 (Huantiao)

GB 1	(Tongziliao)			GB 13	(Benshen)
GB 2	(Tinghu)			GB 14	(Yangbai)
GB 3	(Shangguan)			GB 15	(Linqi)
GB 4	(Hanyan)	GB 8	(Shuaigu)	GB 16	(Muchuang)
GB 5	(Xuanlu)	GB 9	(Tianchong)	GB 17	(Zhengying)
GB 6	(Xuanli)	GB 10	(Fubai)	GB 18	(Chengling)
GB 7	(Qubin)	GB 11	(Qiaogin)	GB 19	(Naong)
		GB 12	(Wangu)	GB 20	(Fengchi)

Points on the Gall Bladder Meridian (GB) – Shaoyang … (1)

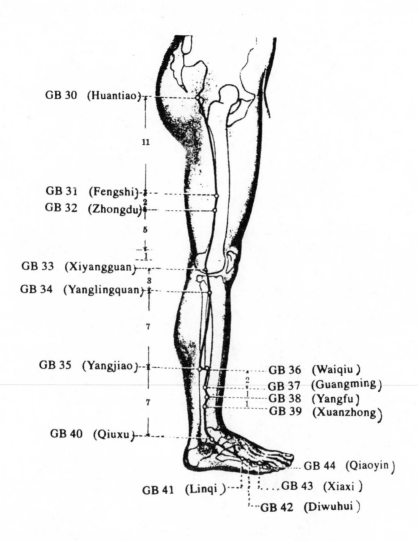

GB 30 (Huantiao)

11

GB 31 (Fengshi)
GB 32 (Zhongdu)
2

5

1

GB 33 (Xiyangguan)
3
GB 34 (Yanglingquan)

7

GB 35 (Yangjiao)
GB 36 (Waiqiu)
2 GB 37 (Guangming)
1 GB 38 (Yangfu)
7 1 GB 39 (Xuanzhong)

GB 40 (Qiuxu)

GB 44 (Qiaoyin)
GB 41 (Linqi)
GB 43 (Xiaxi)
GB 42 (Diwuhui)

Points on the Gall Bladder Meridian (GB) – Shaoyang ... (2)

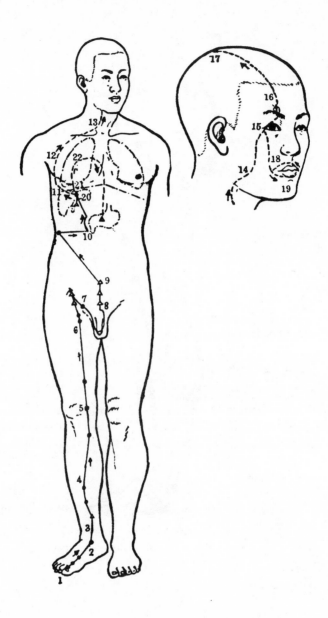

12. Route of the Liver Meridian

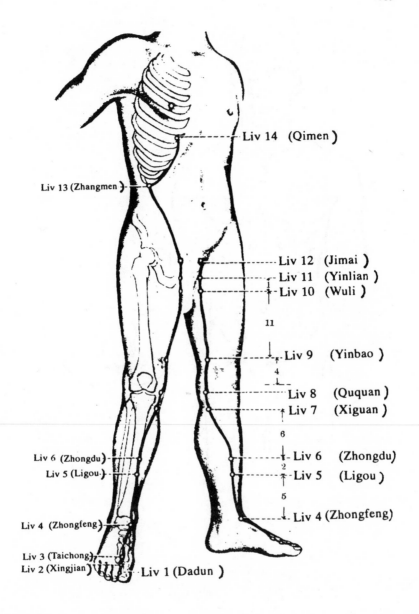

Liv 14 (Qimen)

Liv 13 (Zhangmen)

Liv 12 (Jimai)
Liv 11 (Yinlian)
Liv 10 (Wuli)

11

Liv 9 (Yinbao)

4

Liv 8 (Ququan)
Liv 7 (Xiguan)

6

Liv 6 (Zhongdu)
Liv 5 (Ligou)

Liv 6 (Zhongdu)
Liv 5 (Ligou)

2

5

Liv 4 (Zhongfeng)

Liv 4 (Zhongfeng)

Liv 3 (Taichong)
Liv 2 (Xingjian)
Liv 1 (Dadun)

Points on the Liver Meridian (Liv) – Jueyin

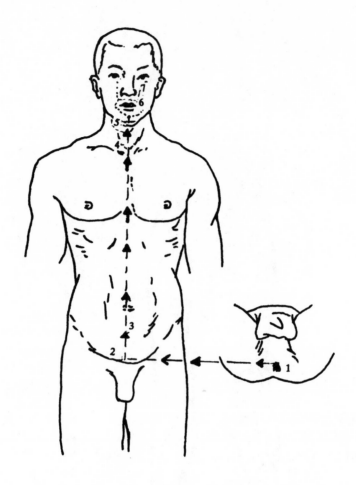

Route of the Conception Vessel Meridian

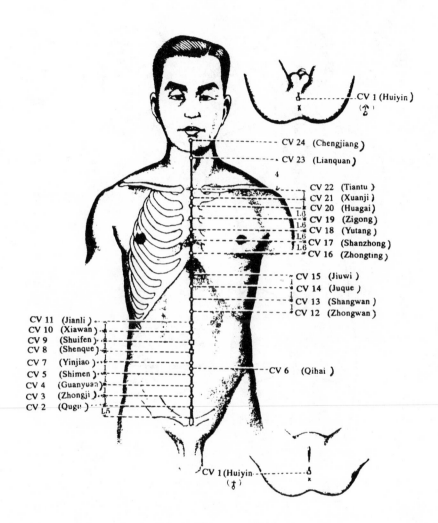

CV 1 (Huiyin)
(♀)

CV 24 (Chengjiang)
CV 23 (Lianquan)

4

CV 22 (Tiantu)
CV 21 (Xuanji)
CV 20 (Huagai)
1.6
CV 19 (Zigong)
1.6
CV 18 (Yutang)
1.6
CV 17 (Shanzhong)
1.6
CV 16 (Zhongting)

CV 15 (Jiuwi)
CV 14 (Juque)
CV 13 (Shangwan)
CV 12 (Zhongwan)

CV 11 (Jianli)
CV 10 (Xiawan)
CV 9 (Shuifen)
CV 8 (Shenque)
CV 7 (Yinjiao)
CV 5 (Shimen)
CV 4 (Guanyuan)
CV 3 (Zhongji)
CV 2 (Qugu)

L5

CV 6 (Qihai)

CV 1 (Huiyin
(♂)

Points on the Conception Vessel Meridian (CV)

472

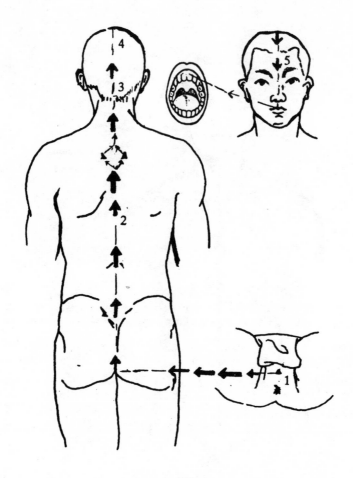

14. Route of the Governor Vessel Meridian

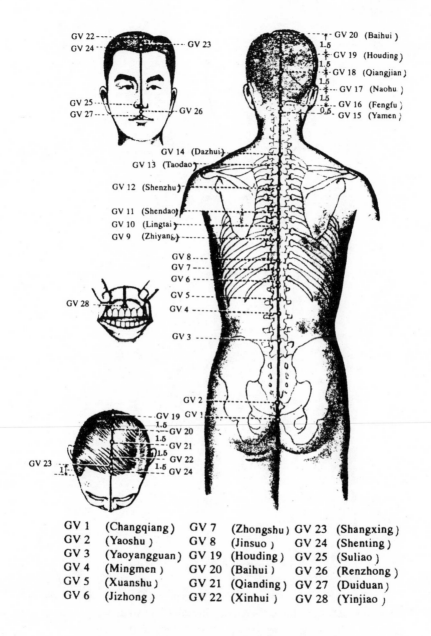

GV 22 --- GV 23
GV 24 ---

GV 20 (Baihui)
1.5
GV 19 (Houding)
1.5
GV 18 (Qiangjian)
1.5
GV 17 (Naohu)
1.5
GV 16 (Fengfu)
0.5
GV 15 (Yamen)

GV 25 ---
GV 27 --- GV 26

GV 14 (Dazhui)
GV 13 (Taodao)
GV 12 (Shenzhu)
GV 11 (Shendao)
GV 10 (Lingtai)
GV 9 (Zhiyang)
GV 8
GV 7
GV 6
GV 5
GV 4
GV 3
GV 2
GV 1

GV 28

GV 19 GV 1
1.5
GV 20
1.5
GV 21
1.5
GV 22
1.5
GV 24
GV 23
1

GV 1	(Changqiang)	GV 7	(Zhongshu)	GV 23	(Shangxing)
GV 2	(Yaoshu)	GV 8	(Jinsuo)	GV 24	(Shenting)
GV 3	(Yaoyangguan)	GV 19	(Houding)	GV 25	(Suliao)
GV 4	(Mingmen)	GV 20	(Baihui)	GV 26	(Renzhong)
GV 5	(Xuanshu)	GV 21	(Qianding)	GV 27	(Duiduan)
GV 6	(Jizhong)	GV 22	(Xinhui)	GV 28	(Yinjiao)

Points on the Governor Vessel Meridian (GV)

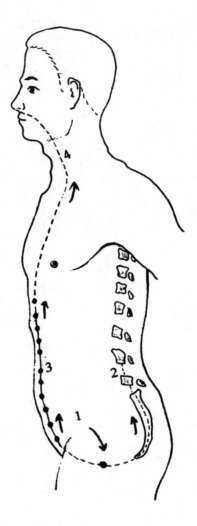

15. Route of the Chong Mo

Starts from the genital and reproductive organs → upwards to the abdomen between the Kidney and Stomach meridians, appropriating points from these two → disperse in the chest → up to the throat → ramifying in the area of the lips.

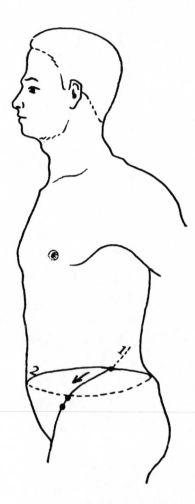

16. Route of the Dai Mo

Starts from the hypochondriac region ➔ running downward around the waist.

476

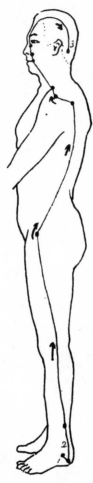

17. Route of the Yangqiao Mo

Starts from the lateral side of the heel ➔ ascending along the
external malleolus ➔ into the external part of the genital organ
➔ upwards along internal part of the abdomen and chest➔ into
Quepan (St 12)➔ ascends along the neck to the corner of the
mouth ➔ enters Jingming (UB 1) and meets with Yinqiao Mo
➔ upward along the UB meridian and meets with GB meridian at
Fengchi (GB 20).

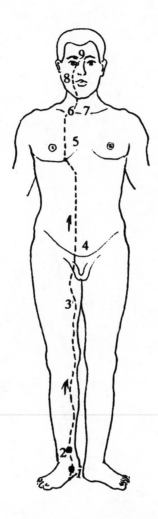

18. Route of the Yinqiao Mo

Starts from the posterior aspect of the navicular bone ➤ ascends
to the upper part of the medial malleolus ➤ upward along leg,
thigh and buttock ➤ to external part of the genital organ ➤ ascends further along the chest ➤ upward lateral to the Renying
(St 9) ➤ into inner canthus (UB 1) and meets with Yangqiao Mo.

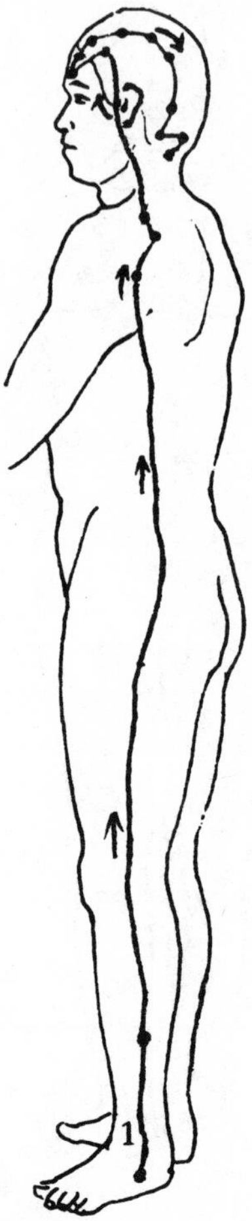

19. Route of the Yangwei Mo

Starts from the heel (UB 63) → ascending to the external malleolus → upward along the GB meridian → passing through the hip → goes up the hypochondriac and costal region → upward along shoulder to the forehead → turns backward to the back of the neck and meets with GV meridian.

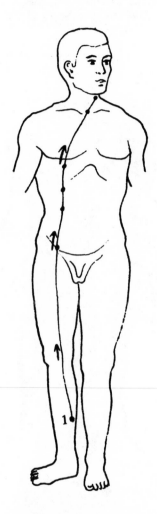

20. Route of the Yinwei Mo

Starts from the medial aspect of the leg (Ki 9) → ascends along
the thigh to the abdomen and meets with the Spleen meridian →
goes up the chest and meets with the CV meridian at the neck (CV
22 and CV 23)

THE CHINESE INCH (CUN)
by BODY LANDMARKS

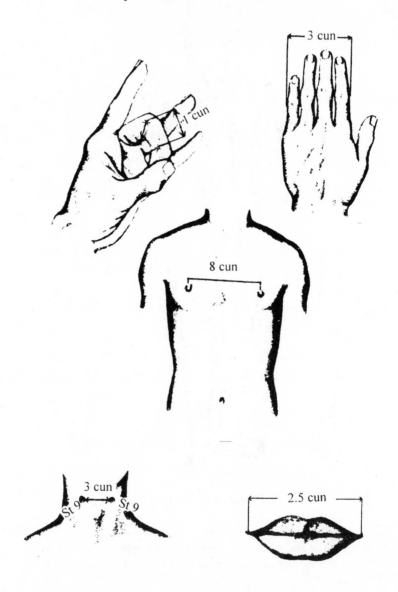

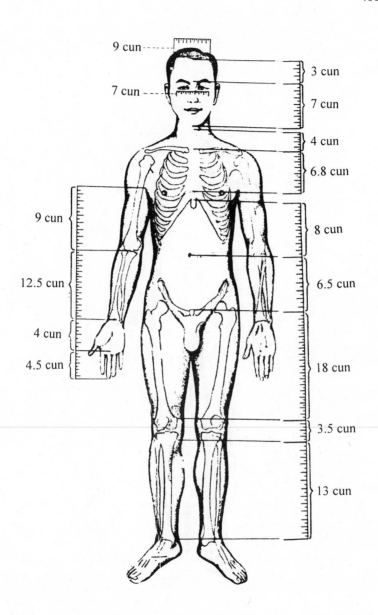

9 cun

7 cun

3 cun

7 cun

4 cun

6.8 cun

9 cun

8 cun

12.5 cun

6.5 cun

4 cun

4.5 cun

18 cun

3.5 cun

13 cun

Frontal View

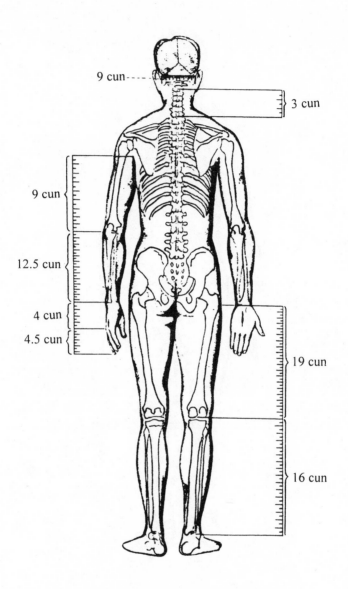

9 cun

3 cun

9 cun

12.5 cun

4 cun

4.5 cun

19 cun

16 cun

Posterior View

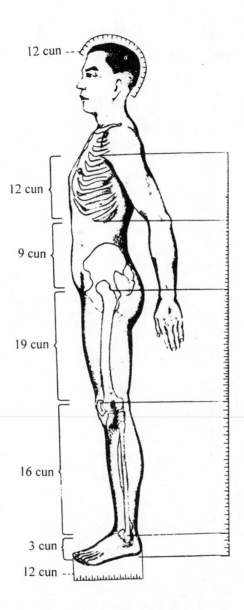

12 cun

12 cun

9 cun

19 cun

16 cun

3 cun

12 cun

Lateral View

484

Timeline of the Valuable Books and Articles in Chinese Medicine

Dynasties

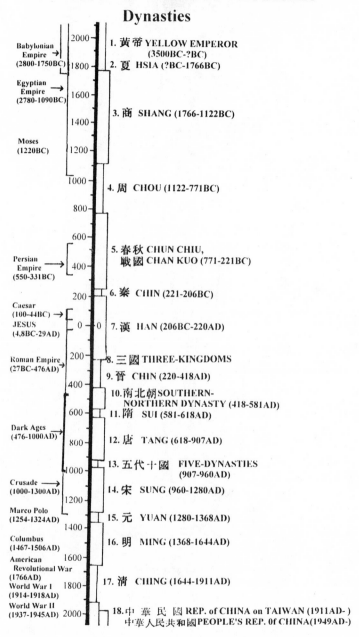

Babylonian Empire → (2800-1750BC)

Egyptian Empire → (2780-1090BC)

Moses (1220BC)

Persian Empire → (550-331BC)

Caesar (100-44BC) →
JESUS (4,8BC-29AD)

Roman Empire → (27BC-476AD)

Dark Ages → (476-1000AD)

Crusade → (1000-1300AD)

Marco Polo (1254-1324AD)

Columbus (1467-1506AD)

American Revolutional War (1766AD)
World War I (1914-1918AD)
World War II (1937-1945AD)

2000
1800
1600
1400
1200
1000
800
600
400
200
0   0
200
400
600
800
1000
1200
1400
1600
1800
2000

1. 黃帝 YELLOW EMPEROR (3500BC-?BC)
2. 夏 HSIA (?BC-1766BC)
3. 商 SHANG (1766-1122BC)
4. 周 CHOU (1122-771BC)
5. 春秋 CHUN CHIU, 戰國 CHAN KUO (771-221BC)
6. 秦 CHIN (221-206BC)
7. 漢 HAN (206BC-220AD)
8. 三國 THREE-KINGDOMS
9. 晉 CHIN (220-418AD)
10. 南北朝 SOUTHERN-NORTHERN DYNASTY (418-581AD)
11. 隋 SUI (581-618AD)
12. 唐 TANG (618-907AD)
13. 五代十國 FIVE-DYNASTIES (907-960AD)
14. 宋 SUNG (960-1280AD)
15. 元 YUAN (1280-1368AD)
16. 明 MING (1368-1644AD)
17. 清 CHING (1644-1911AD)
18. 中華民國 REP. of CHINA on TAIWAN (1911AD-)
中華人民共和國 PEOPLE'S REP. 0f CHINA (1949AD-)

Valuable Books and Articles

→ 1, 2, 3

內 經 Nei Jing
(Yellow Emperor's Inner Canon)

- Created Chinese medicine
- Stone and bone needles were utilized
  for the first time

→ 4

山 海 經 San Hai Jing
(Montain & Sea Canon for Herbal medicine)

- 扁 鵲 (Ben Her)- The most famous
  acupuncture doctor in the history

→ 5

難 經 Nan Jing
(Canon of Perplexities)
參 同 契 Zsen Tong Chi
(The Kinship of the Three)

- Confucius (551-478BC)

→ 6

呂氏春秋 Lee Shi Chun Chu,
Lee Bu-Wei (215BC)
(Lee's Spring and Autumn Annals for
Principle of Chinese medicine)

- Built Great Wall

→ 7

傷 論 Sang Han Lun, Chang Chun-
寒 Jan (204AD)
(Treatise on Injury by Cold)
淮南子 Huai Nan Zi, Lu An (122BC)
(Theory of Chinese medicine)
金匱要略 Jin Kui Yao Lue, Chang
Ji (220AD)
(Prescriptions of the Golden
Chamber)

- Buddhism and Indian medicine
  introduced in China
- 華 佗 HwaTou (112-207AD)- The
  most famous doctor of Chinese
  medicine in the history

→ 8, 9

脈 經 Mai Jing, Wang Shu-Her (302AD)
(Canon of Pulse Diagnosis)

→ 10

甲 乙經 Jia Yi Jing, Huang Fu-Mi (282AD)
(Systematic Canon of Acupuncture and
Moxibustion)

- Chinese Medicine introduced into
  Korea (541AD) and Japan (562AD)

→ 11

諸 源候論 Zhu Bing Yuan Hou Lun, Chao
病 Yan-Fang (610AD)
(Treatise on the Cause and Effect of
Disorders)
黃 內經太素 Huang Di Nei Jing Tai Su,
帝 Yang Shan-Shan (607AD)
(Yellow Emperor's Inner Cannon)
古 今錄驗方 Ku Chin Lu Ehn Fun (618-
626AD)
(Prescriptions of the Ancient and modern
times)

486

→ 12   素 釋
黃帝內經文問 Huang Di Nei Jing Shu
Wen Su Wen, Wang Ben (762AD)
(Yellow Emperor's Inner Canon, Interpreted
and Explained)
千金方 Chian Jin Fun, Sun Si-Mo (652AD)
(Numerous and Valued Prescriptions)
- Estabolished Doctoral degree in Chinese
  medicine

→ 13
- A prosperous perior for literary works of
  clinical Chinese medicine

→ 14
銅人經 Tong Ren Jing, Wang Wei Yi (1026AD)
(Illustrated Canon of Bronze Statue
Acupuncture Points)

→ 15
針灸四方 Zhen Jiu Si Fun, Dou Gui-Fang
(1311AD)
(Four Essential Books of Acupuncture and
Moxibustion)
難經本義 Nan Jing Ben Yi, Hua Shou
(1361AD)
(Essential Meaning of the Canon Perplexities)

→ 16
針灸大成 Zhen Jiu Da Chun, Yang Da-Chou
(1601AD)
(Collection of Acupuncture and Moxibustion)
針灸聚英 Zhen Jiu Ju En, Gao Wu (1546AD)
(An Essential gathering of Acupuncture and
Moxibustion)
醫學入門 Yi Xue Zu Men, Lee Chan
(1575AD)
(Gateway to Chinese medicine)
類經 Lei Jing, Chang Jie-Bin (1624AD)
(Canon of Categories)
本草綱目 Been Cao Kang Moon, Lee
Shi-Jin (1578AD)
(The Listed Medicinal Plants and Animals)

→ 17
傷寒續論 Shang Han Shu Lu, Chang Lu
(1669 AD)
(Treatise on Injury by Cold- Advanced
Interpretation)
難經經解 Nan Jing Jing Jie,Hsu Da -Tzun
(1727AD)
(Explanation of the Canon of Perplexities)
血證論 Xue Zheng Lun, Tang Zhong-Hai
(1885AD)
(A Theory on the Differential Diagnosis of
Blood)
難經正義 Nan Jing Zheng Yi, Yee Lin
(1895AD)
(Appropriate Meaning of the Canon of
Perplexities)

BIBLIOGRAPHY

1. Acupuncture and Science, Chinese edition: Chou Zi- Hua, Chi Ye Publishing Co., Taipei, 1977

2. Anatomy and Physiology of the Inner Canon, Chinese edition: National Chinese Medical Research Bureau, Taipei, 1965

3. Classics of Acupuncture, Chinese edition: Yang Wei - Ji, Lo Chin Publishing Co., Taipei, 1975

4. Compendium of Scalp Acupuncture, Chinese edition: Yang Wei - Ji, Lo Chin Publishing Co., Taipei, 1975

5. Compendium of Secret Prescription of Chinese Medicine, Chinese edition: Teh Shen Publishing Co., Taipei, 1982

6. Diagnosis of Chinese Acupuncture, Chinese edition: Ma Jin - Chong, National Publishing Bureau, Taipei, 1982

7. Essential of Chinese Acupuncture, Chinese - English edition: People's Health Press, Beijing, 1978

8. Essential Meaning of the Canon of Perplexities, Chinese edition; Xuan Feng Publishing Co. Taipei, 1979

9. Interpretation of Difficult Part of Acupuncture and Moxibustion, Chinese edition: Chi Ye Publishing Co., Taipei, 1987

10. Nan Jing (Canon of Perplexities), Chinese edition: Found in Wang Shu - He (A. D. 300)

11. National Symposia of Acupuncture and Moxibustion and Acupuncture Anesthesia, English edition: Research Group of Acupuncture, Beijing, 1979

12. Physician's Handbook, Chinese edition: Tsay, Kuen - Shii, Shen Lou Publishing Co., Taipei, 1979

13. Practical Acupuncture Prescribing Method, Chinese edition: Wu Chi - Lian, Ruey Shen Publishing Co. Taipei, 1988

14. Priceless Prescriptions, Chinese edition: Sun Si - Mo (A. D. 652) National Chinese Medical Herb Research Center, Taipei, 1980

15. Shan Han Lun (Treatise on Injury by Cold and Heat), Chinese edition: Zhang Ji (A. D. 220), National Chinese Medical Research Bureau, Taipei, 1965

16. The Johns Hopkins Atlas of Human Functional Anatomy, English edition: George D. Zuidema, The Johns Hopkins University School of Medicine, 1982

17. The Methodology of Acupuncture and Moxibustion, Chinese edition: Xi Yung - Jiang, Shanghai, 1985

18. The Pressure Pain Point in Acupuncture, English edition: Chung C., Veterans General Hospital, Taipei, 1983

19. The Secret Prescription of A Great Doctor - Hua To, Chinese edition: Hua To - Shen, Huan yee Publishing Co., Taipei,1972

20. Treatise on the Origin and Outcome of Disease: Chinese edition: Chao Yan - Fang
(A. D. 610), National Chinese Medical Pharmacology Research Group, Beijing, 1984

Index

A

B

C

490

Irregular menstruation
113, 114, 116, 117, 118, 253, 297, 401

J

Jianchian 147
Jianho 147
Jing Luo 49
Jing-River Points 163
Jing-Well Points 162, 166
Jueyin 151, 154
Jueyin Syndrome 97, 102

K

Kidney 62, 72
Kidney Deficiency 36
Kidney Meridian (Ki) 114
Kidney Yang 114
Kidney Yin 114
Knee Tri-Needle 303
KONG ZUI/Lu 6 137
KUN LUN/ UB 60 131
Kunlun (UB 60) through to Taixi (Ki 3) 287

L

Large Intestine Meridian (L.I.) 109
Leukorrhea 116, 117, 118, 297, 401
LIANG QUI/St 34 125
LIE QUE/Lu 7 137
Lift and Thrust Method 236
Liver 61, 67
Liver fire 116
Liver Fire Ascending 68, 69
Liver Meridian (Liv) 116
Liver Qi
    Depression of 67
        Clinical signs and symptoms 68
        Disharmony 68
Liver Wind 70
Liver Yang Ascending 69
Liver-gall bladder region 348
Lobule 362, 365, 369, 378
Local Hematoma 226
Location of Auricular Points 366
Lower Abdominal Tri-Needle 297
Lower He Sea Points 190

Lower jiao 50
Lumbar Tri-Needle 300
Lung 61, 65
Lung Meridian (Lu) 109
Luo points 177, 193
Lymphangitis 228

M

Manipulation Methods for Tonification and Dispersion 390
Manipulation of the Needle 214
Mark lines of scalp acupuncture 334
Menorrhagia 111, 116, 117, 130, 311
Menostasia 117
Mental confusion 146
Mernier's syndrome 340
Method of imbedding needles 392
Method of Needle Insertion 352, 389
Methods for Point Prescription 143
Methods of Application 416
Middle jiao 50
Migraine headache 115, 116, 144
Most Commonly Used Points 121
Most important points 121
Mother and Son Points 168
Motor Region 335
Motorial epilepsy 340
Move Qi 315
Moving Qi Method 261
Moving Qi method 262
Moxa 413
Moxa Instrument 419
Moxa pole 418
Moxa stick 309, 311
Moxa Sticks 417
Moxa wool 413
MOXIBUSTION 413
Moxibustion 413
Mu Points 190
Muscular atrophy 253

N

Nasal bleeding 144, 147
Neck stiffness 144
Neck Tri-Needle 293
Needle Sensation 355
Needle Stimulation 215
NEI GUAN/ Pc 6 124
Nei Jing 361, 404

Z